Diabetic Keto Diet:

Keto Diet Plan for Diabetes. Diabetic Keto Cookbook.

by

Viktoria McCartney

Text Copyright [Viktoria McCartney]

All rights reserved. No part of this guide may be reproduced in any form without permission in writing from the publisher except in the case of brief quotations embodied in critical articles or reviews.

Table of Contents

Introduction 6

How Having a Keto Diet Reduces the Risk of Developing Diabetes Type 2 8

Understanding a Keto Diet 10

General Guide when Choosing Food to Eat 11

Foods to Avoid 24

Diabetic Plate Recipes 29

Chicken and Turkey Recipes 30

   Pumpkin, Bean, and Chicken Enchiladas 30

   Mu Shu Chicken 33

   Stove-Top Chicken, Macaroni, and Cheese 35

   Chicken Sausage Omelets with Spinach 37

   Chicken-Broccoli Salad with Buttermilk Dressing 39

   Country-Style Wedge Salad with Turkey 41

   Turkey Kabob Pitas 43

Beef and Lamb Recipes 46

   Spicy Beef Sloppy Joes 46

   Roasted Steak and Tomato Salad 48

   Lamb Fatteh with Asparagus 50

   Beef Goulash Soup 52

   Beef-Vegetable Ragout 54

   Greek Flat Iron Steaks 56

    Spiced Burgers with Cilantro Cucumber Sauce 58

Fish and Seafood Recipes **60**

    Caribbean Fish with Mango-Orange Relish 60

    Lemon-Herb Roasted Salmon Sheet-Pan Dinner 62

    Shrimp and Chicken Dumpling Soup 64

    Cod with Eggplant Peperonata 66

    Parmesan-Crusted Cod with Garlicky Summer Squash 68

    Fried Cauliflower Rice with Shrimp 70

    Quick Scallop and Noodle Toss 72

Meatless/Vegan Recipes **74**

    Falafel and Vegetable Pitas 74

    Chickpea Alfredo with Spring Veggies 77

    Mediterranean Fried Quinoa 79

    Asparagus and Greens with Farro 81

    Toasted Walnut Tempeh Tacos 83

    Mushroom-Lentil Shepard's Pie 85

    Sesame-Mustard Oats with Charred Green Onions 88

Desserts **90**

    Frozen Yogurt Bark 90

    Sweet Ricotta and Strawberry Parfaits 92

    Chocolate-Date Truffles 94

    Citrus Custard 96

    Creamy Chocolate Pudding 98

    Peanut Butter Butterscotch Bites 100

Apricot Pocket Cookies.. 102
Conclusion 105

Introduction

Diabetes type 2 is the cells inability to respond to insulin or the pancreatic cells not being able to produce enough insulin. So how does each of these conditions occur? For whatever reason, if your pancreas is not producing enough insulin and you continue to eat high carb sugary meals, the little insulin that was produced will not be able to drop the high blood glucose levels back to normal after meals.

As a result, the pancreas cells will still detect high blood glucose levels and will try to produce more and more insulin. However, the pancreas has a production capacity of a certain amount, but the constant stimulation causes it to try and exceed its production capacity of insulin. Eventually, this leads to the exhaustion of the pancreatic cells. When this happens after every meal that is loaded with sugars day after day, the pancreatic cells eventually wear out and can become permanently damaged. Though they mostly only become temporarily damaged and return to their normal state when the glucose stress subsides. <u>That is why lowering blood glucose via eating a low carb diet or exercising is an effective strategy to reverse and manage diabetes type 2.</u>

The second issue regarding eating high carb meals is that you are producing lots of insulin in order to be able to bring the glucose levels back to normal. The excessive exposure to insulin desensitizes the cells and makes them unresponsive to insulin.

When the cells lose their sensitivity to insulin, they become unable to respond to the signal of insulin that triggers cells to remove glucose from the blood. As a result, when the cells develop insulin insensitivity, no matter how much insulin is produced, the blood will still have increased levels of glucose. As a result, the pancreatic cells are still affecting high glucose levels and are trying to produce more and more insulin. As you see, this results in a vicious cycle, exhausting the pancreatic cells and increasing the insulin insensitivity of the cells. When your pancreatic cells are exhausted, you can no longer produce insulin, and if insulin is produced, it is produced in very low and insufficient amounts which further contributes to developing diabetes type 2. <u>Following a low carb diet can help you decrease the risk of developing diabetes type 2.</u>

How Having a Keto Diet Reduces the Risk of Developing Diabetes Type 2

When you minimize your intake of sugars and carbohydrates, you shift your metabolism into a healthier alternative that decreases your risk factors of developing diabetes type 2.

To begin with, having a reduced intake of carbohydrates and sugar means you decrease the body's need to release insulin in large quantities. This has a twofold benefit as it protects your pancreatic cells from exhaustion as they no longer need to secrete insulin in crazy amounts to restore your rising blood glucose levels. Moreover, it prevents insulin insensitivity from occurring as your cells are not exposed to large amounts of insulin frequently.

Other benefits of reducing your carb intake is that you are going to lose weight. Being overweight is a risk factor for developing diabetes. An additional fact is that too much insulin relates to weight gain.

Insulin in nature is an anabolic hormone. That means it causes the macromolecules to be built. Macromolecules are molecules such as fats and carbohydrates. So, in other words, insulin causes fats to be built rather than broken down, and this is the opposite of losing weight. This is in fact how you gain weight.

Additionally, your body uses mainly glucose for respiration. However, you can shift the molecule that your body uses for respiration and cause your body to burn fat rather than glucose. However, when there is an abundance of glucose available, your body will always be burning glucose and will leave fats alone.

Fat molecules in the presence of insulin, the anabolic hormone, will be built up and stored. This leads to the accumulation of fat around your organs and under your skin leaving you to gain weight overall. Weight gain further makes you lazy to exercise or carry on a physically active lifestyle, further increasing your risk of developing or worsening your diabetes.

The fats can also accumulate in your arteries and near your heart, leading you to have atherosclerosis, which is a condition that increases your risk of cardiovascular diseases and predisposes you to develop hypertension. So overall, simple and healthy habits such as having predominantly high carbohydrates and high in sugar diet can lead to a cascade of disorders including aggravating diabetes type 2 and increasing your risk of developing diabetes if you didn't have t; as well as increasing your risk of developing cardiac disorders.

Understanding a Keto Diet

The definition of a keto diet is one that has very little carbohydrates. There are many types of low carb diets but the ones that proved to be beneficial to managing diabetes, substituted the carbs with a source of healthy fats. That way, it becomes a low carb, high-fat diet. If you are going to cut the carbs, you need to provide your body with an alternative source of energy. In this case, it is healthy fats.

That means greatly minimizing or cutting out foods that are high in starch and carbs such as rice, pasta, processed sugary foods, foods containing flour like white bread, etc. While loading up your diet with high fiber and low glycemic index foods such as vegetables, healthy fats and proteins to a lesser extent.

In addition to managing your diabetes, a keto diet is a healthy way to lose weight and promote your overall health. It converts your body from being a sugar burning machine into a fat burning machine. However, note that there is a transition period of about 7 to 14 days before your body successfully and completely switches from burning sugars to burning fats. During this transition period, your body will suffer from mild changes due to the deprivation of carbs (remember, it still depends on carbs during the transition period).

General Guide when Choosing Food to Eat

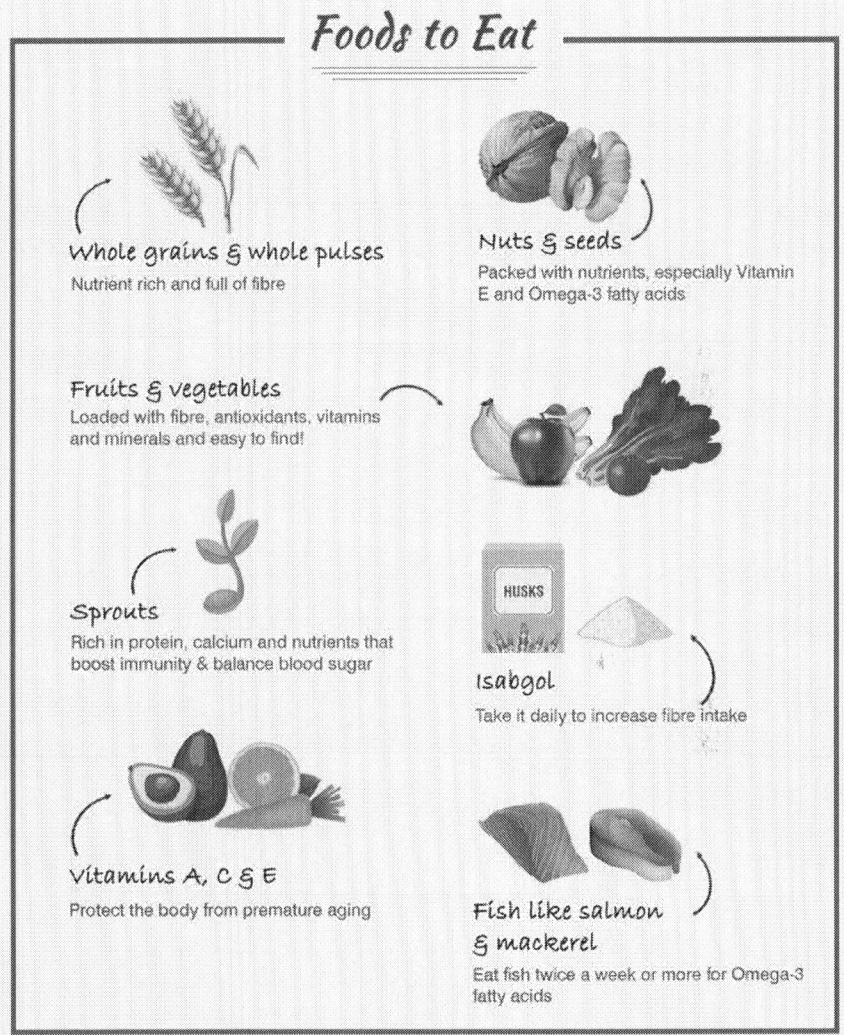

No matter what kind of diet you are attempting to follow, it is not correct to completely eliminate an entire food group. While in diabetes there are certain food groups that you can try to minimize your intake of such as starch and sugars but don't fall prey to the mistake of completely eliminating starch as your body needs carbs. Instead, what you must do is to choose wisely between the various food options in each category to ensure that you ingest the best and most suitable food type from each category and avoid the ones that will worsen your condition.

The goal of controlling your food with diabetes is eating food that will not increase your blood glucose levels higher than normal. At the same time it needs to be food that makes you feel full and keeps hunger at bay; in addition, certain food categories can promote your health and provide you with nutritional elements that can help you fight off diabetes and protect you from its complications.

It is important to note that there is no one-size-fits-all when it comes to healthy eating plans for diabetic patients. There are lots of personal variations in the way our body responds to nutrition and different food intake styles however there are general rules that can be observed if you have diabetes and wish to control your blood sugar and keep its complications at bay.

Low Starch Food

Whole grains for example, oatmeal, quinoa and brown rice are preferred and healthier than white rice, white flour or processed grains, macaroni, etc.

Baked sweet potato provides a low carb option in contrast to regular potato such as French fries. Other items that contain high carbs include white bread and white flour etc. Instead, opt for whole grain foods that have very little added sugar or not at all.

Non-Starchy Vegetables

One of the healthiest options if you're diabetic is to include a couple of servings of non-starchy vegetables per day. There is very little chance that you could go wrong with overeating non-starchy vegetables, that is because they have a very low calorific intake.

Non starchy vegetables are vegetables that contain a small amount of carbohydrate. This is typically about 5 grams or less of carbohydrate per a 100g of serving. It is recommended by the American Diabetes Association that you have your plate half-filled with non-starchy vegetables.

Throughout your day, it should be your goal that you have at least five portions of fruit and vegetables and out of those 5, it is best to have at least three of them that are non-starchy vegetables.

There are several reasons why non-starchy vegetables are a very healthy options for diabetics. The foremost reason is that they are very low in carbs. Other reasons include how non-starchy vegetables are very nutritious. They are full of vitamins and minerals as well as other critical nutrients such as phytochemicals. In addition, being vegetables, they are a critical source of dietary fiber. The dietary fiber will help you to digest food properly and it also plays an important role in lowering your cholesterol levels. Overall, dietary fiber is an essential nutrient to include in your diet.

Non-starchy vegetables are a very powerful defense against the complications of diabetes. They help to protect your cells from the damage induced by the disorder of diabetes and promote the health of your blood vessels which can also be compromised during the course of diabetes progression.

Non-starchy vegetables are also rich in vitamins and minerals such as vitamin A, vitamin C and vitamin K. Vitamin C helps to promote your immunity and protect your cells from oxidative damage.

A good source of non-starchy vegetables containing vitamin C are peppers, sprouts and broccoli. You can easily add peppers to your salad or main dish. Steamed broccoli is also a very healthy option to add to your main dish or serve alongside salmon or to add to your veggie pan salad.

Vitamin E is also helpful in boosting your immune system; it is also important for your eye health as well as for your skin. Carrots, kale and spinach are options rich in vitamin E that you can easily add them to your food.

Vitamin K is going to assist in wound healing and improving health as well as preventing atherosclerosis. Diabetics are at risk of atherosclerosis if they have uncontrolled diabetes. Moreover, they have poor wound healing so food rich in vitamin K such as green leafy vegetables will help promote the health of diabetics and prevent infections as a result of poor wound healing.

Below are Some Examples of Non-Starchy Vegetables

Leafy vegetables: kale, lettuce, spinach, watercress, cabbage, Brussel sprouts.

Root vegetables: carrot, turnip, radishes.

Squashes: cucumber, squash, courgette, pumpkin.

Stalk vegetables: asparagus, leeks, spring onions, celery.

Others: broccoli, bean sprouts, mushroom, cauliflower, peppers, tomato.

As a diabetic, vegetables are your best friend. Fresh vegetables when eaten raw or even when steamed, roasted or grilled, can be a very healthy low carb option. The same applies to frozen vegetables that are lightly steamed. Always opt for low sodium or unsalted canned vegetables. Canned vegetables with lots of added sodium are not a healthy option.

Also, it is counterproductive if you eat veggies that are cooked with lots of butter cheese or a high carb source. If you are having hypertension or other complications of diabetes and metabolic syndrome then you need to limit your intake of sodium and that includes limiting pickles etc.

Fatty Fish

Examples: Herring, Salmon anchovies, mackerel, sardine.

Fatty fish are one of the most consistent diet recommendations when it comes to fending off diseases. Diabetes is no exception. Fish is one of the most beneficial foods you can eat if you have diabetes.

Since having diabetes poses a risk on your heart functions it is important to take cardioprotective measures. Salmon contains Omega-3 fatty acids which have a profound positive effect on your heart health. Taking care and promoting your heart health helps against the increased risk of heart disease and stroke that people with diabetes are faced with. In addition, studies have shown that several inflammatory markers had dropped when fatty fish was consumed 5 to 7 days per week for about 8 weeks. In addition to all that it contains high quality protein and is low in carbs, therefore, is perfect for maintaining normal blood glucose sugars after meals.

Dairy

Dairy food is an important food category and with a variety of choices available for you to pick from. Studies have shown that milk product consumption and total dairy products have been associated with a reduced risk of developing type 2 diabetes. It is also protective for those who have prediabetes. The mechanisms explaining this evidence is complicated but simply put, certain biomarker fatty acids found in dairy milk are associated with lowering the risk of developing diabetes type 2. The studies were conducted on each of the following items from the dairy group including whole milk and yoghurt in addition to total dairy consumption.

Examples of dairy food include milk, yoghurt, cream, butter and cheese. Unsweetened dairy products can be a very healthy choice for those who wish to follow a low-carb diet. There are numerous benefits for dairy foods as they are a good source of protein, calcium and vitamin B12. It is recommended by the National Osteoporosis Society that a daily intake of 700 mg of calcium is required for adults to maintain healthy bones as well as other functions that depend on calcium.

Vitamin B12 is an important source for the nervous system. Diabetics are at risk of complications of neuropathy that affects the peripheral nerves. Vitamin B12 helps protect against some of the complications of diabetes concerning the nerves. The protein in milk is also important for muscle repair and growth. The recommended daily intake of calcium can be achieved by just a pint of milk along with another source that includes food such as beans, fish with edible bones such as sardines and salmon and dark green vegetables, for example, kale and broccoli.

For dairy opt for low-fat dairy if you want to have high fat or full fat dairy do so but in small proportions. The best choices are skimmed milk, low-fat yoghurt and low-fat or non-fat sour cream or cottage cheese. Some of the worst choices are whole milk, regular yoghurt, regular sour cream, cottage cheese and ice cream etc.

Beans and Pulses

Beans, pulses: lentils peas chickpeas and runner beans are all examples of non-animal sources of protein that can be very beneficial for diabetics.

Soya Beans have been included among this group and it has been supported with research indicating that the consumption of soya beans increases insulin sensitivity and reduces the risk of developing type 2 diabetes. In fact, certain countries in Asia have been using black soya beans to combat type 2 diabetes.

Adding beans to your salads is a good option for increasing your protein intake.

Fruits

Just like vegetables, fruits are one of the healthiest food groups that you can add to your diet. They are rich in nutrients especially vitamin C which helps to keep your cells healthy. In addition to the minerals, we also have fiber which help digestion, and it reduces cholesterol levels. Different fruits have a different combination of vitamins and minerals; for example, grapefruits can be rich in vitamin A as well as potassium; they can also be rich in vitamin K and manganese. A meta-analysis showed that groups of people who consumed higher amount of fruits were at less risk of developing type 2 diabetes.

It is recommended by the American Diabetes Association to use fruits as a dessert option rather than having a sugar-loaded desserts such as ice cream. While fruits have dense nutrients as well as fiber and antioxidants it is important to remember that certain foods have a high glycemic index and can increase your blood sugar levels, therefore, it is important to be mindful about the types of fruits you eat and when.

Bananas and oranges are fruits that have high glycemic index while berries for example or less sugary.

Below are some examples of <u>fruits that have a glycemic index of under 55</u>:

Grapefruit, grapes, kiwi, apples, avocados, peaches, plums strawberries.

<u>Fruit with medium glycemic index from 56 to 69</u>:

Pineapples, papayas, honeydew melon.

<u>Foods with high glycemic index that is more than 70</u>:

Watermelon and dates.

Avoid processed foods such as apple sauce that have had their fiber removed. if you have a sweet tooth, fruits can be an optimum way to satisfy your desires without compromising your health. Since fruits are high in nutrients and low in fat and sodium, they are optimum if you have obesity or hypertension.

One serving of fruit is a medium-sized fruit that is the size of the piece. Or a cup of smaller fruits such as berries. So, you should avoid it, but if you have processed fruits have only half a cup of processed fruits to fulfil the serving size.

Apples. An apple is a versatile fruit that you can snack on raw or cook it with some flavoring such as cinnamon or ginger to make a delicious dessert. You can also stuff your apples with some crushed nuts such as walnuts or pecans.

Avocados. Avocados are very high in healthy fats which are the Mono- unsaturated fats that are beneficial to your body. Avocados are a tasty option to add to your main dish; slice along with some salmon or make guacamole. They're very easy to prepare or include in any of your dishes.

Berries. Berries are a very delicious and versatile fruit. There are strawberries, blueberries, blackberries, etc. There are a lot of things that you can do with berries, for example, you can eat them raw or you can make them into a smoothie. You can always add various berries to most of your breakfast or snacks, for example, making an oatmeal breakfast or adding various to your fresh whipped cream or frozen yoghurt. They are also rich in antioxidants and very low on calories. They help fight inflammation and other diseases such as cancer.

Citrus fruits. They are also good for boosting your immunity; they are loaded with vitamin C. One orange contains all the amount of vitamin c that you require in a day. Since immunity is an issue with diabetics adding citrus foods to your diet is very healthy and useful low carb option. You can add lemons to your seafood or sauces or even to your iced water or tea. You can simply make lemons or oranges into a refreshing cold drink. The folate and potassium in oranges help you to equalize your blood pressure if you suffer from hypertension. Citrus foods also include grapefruits as well as oranges and lemons.

Peaches. They are juicy and delicious fragrant foods that contain lots of nutrients such as vitamins A and C as well as fiber and minerals such as potassium. They are easy to add in your yoghurt or spice them up with some cinnamon or ginger. You can also flavor your tea with peach instead of sugar for a healthy twist on your drinks.

Pears. They are also a tasty treat that you can add up to your salad or snack on. They are rich in fiber and are a good source of vitamin K.

Kiwi is a slightly citrus fruit that is rich in fiber and vitamin C as well as potassium. One large kiwi contains about 13 grams of carbohydrates which is low carb, making it a delicious yet very healthy option to add to your diet.

Lean Meat

A source of protein that is low in fat and low in calorie is lean meat. That means the red meat such as pork chops that are trimmed of fat or skinless chicken or turkey.

A nutritional source of protein for promoting cell health and repair is lean meat while also being a low carb and low-fat option. Poultry is also a rich source of vitamin B3, B6 choline and selenium. Vitamin B3 which is known as niacin helps with stress and sex hormones. Erectile dysfunction and stress are an issue for those who have diabetes and having food with vitamin B3 become very beneficial for diabetics. Niacin helps with promoting the function of nerves and can reduce inflammation. Selenium has strong antioxidant properties that help with controlling inflammation and protecting the cells. Selenium also has a function in promoting the immune system which is very beneficial for people with diabetes.

Red meat is also a rich source of protein, iron, zinc and vitamin B. Iron is important for your red blood cells, to transport oxygen, as healthy cells require a constant supply of oxygen. Anemia which is a deficiency in RBCs can occur due to a deficiency in iron which is a condition that could easily be avoided by eating adequate amounts of iron. Iron can also be found in dark green leafy plants, as well as beans, iron from greens is the best source.

Zinc is also a mineral needed by the body for the synthesis of DNA. It also has a role in helping the immune system to function properly. You can also find zinc in fish eggs as well as beans, although zinc is better absorbed from fish and meat sources.

Red meat is rich in vitamin B6 and B12. Both are helpful for promoting the immune system, regeneration and protection of the nervous system. One medication that some diabetics take is known as metformin causes an increased drop in vitamin B12. Therefore, it becomes necessary to compensate for the loss of vitamin B from sources such as red meat.

Eggs

Be mindful about the number of eggs you consume as they can easily raise your cholesterol levels. If you're going to eat an egg, it is preferred that it's boiled and consume the whole egg as the benefits of eggs lines in the nutrients inside, rather than the whites. It is a debate whether eggs are helpful or not for diabetics due to due to their low carb content; however, consuming an excessive amount of eggs is associated with the risk of increasing cholesterol levels. Moreover, apart from being rich in cholesterol, eggs are dense in nutrients as they have essential fatty acids proteins and vitamin D.

Nuts

Studies have found that nuts help to decrease the risk of developing type 2 diabetes the *Journal of the American College of Nutrition* stated that consumption of nuts is associated with decreasing the prevalence of certain risk factors that are associated with developing type 2 diabetes and other metabolic disorders. Some have more benefits than other, for example, almonds are rich in nutrients particularly vitamin E. Cashews contain a lot of magnesium. Almonds, cashews and peanuts are nuts that help to reduce the bad cholesterol. Walnuts are rich in Omega-3 fatty acids

Nuts that work on reducing the bad cholesterol are very effective because they protect diabetics from the complication of the narrowing of arteries.

Cashews. Consuming cashews is very beneficial to lower your blood pressure and decrease the risk of heart disease and therefore reduce the risk of getting diabetes type 2. They are also low in calories; therefore, they have no negative effect on your blood glucose level. They are also low in fat, so they do not affect your weight negatively. You can have about a handful of cashews every day for the maximum benefit.

Peanuts. Peanuts are rich in fiber and protein, and therefore they are a beneficial option for people suffering from diabetes. You can have up to 25 to 30 peanuts every day. You can also roast them. They have the ability to control your blood glucose levels.

Pistachios. They are loaded with energy however they are good sources of protein and a good source of healthy fats which can make you feel full for a long time, therefore, curbing the urge to snack. A study performed showed that eating pistachios was very beneficial for people suffering from diabetes. Avoid salted pistachios however.

Walnuts are high in calories; however, they do not affect your body weight. They have numerous nutritional benefits and consuming walnuts daily can help in weight loss due to their low carbohydrate content and their possession of substances that activate the fat burning pathways. They also educe fasting glucose, which help you avoid obesity as a complication of diabetes. The high calorie content helps your body by providing it with energy so that you don't feel like eating a lot and therefore gain weight.

Almonds control the blood glucose level and are very beneficial for diabetics because they help to reduce the oxidative stress which affects cells in diabetics. They are also rich in magnesium. Avoid salted almonds, and you can also soak them in water overnight to eat them fresh the next day.

Foods to Avoid

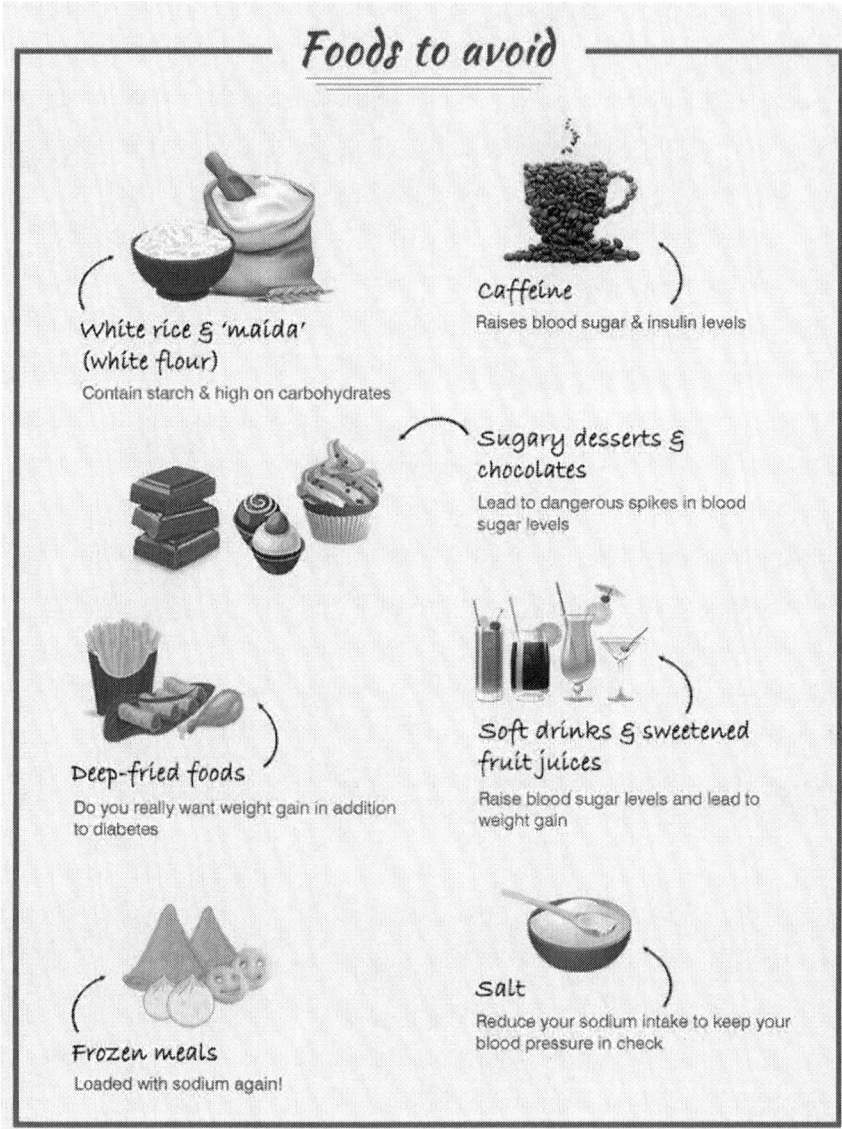

Beverages that are sweetened with sugar

These beverages are some of the worst choices to obtain for diabetics. This is because they are very high in carbs. For example, a 12 oz can of soda has roughly 38 grams of carbs. The same applies for sweetened iced tea or sweetened lemonade as they contain about 35 g of carbs per serving.

Moreover, these sweetened drinks are full of fructose which has been strongly associated with increased insulin resistance and worsening of diabetes. On top of promoting diabetes, high levels of fructose also results in having belly fat and leads to the build-up of harmful cholesterol and increases the level of triglycerides. This shift in metabolism will not help to control your diabetes.

Trans fats

These are fats that are made by adding hydrogen to unsaturated fatty acids in order to stabilize them. Examples of trans fats can be found in margarine and frozen dinners. In addition, many food companies add trans fats to the muffins and baked goods to give them a better taste and extend their expiry date.

Trans fats do not have a direct effect on raising your blood glucose levels, however, they increase your insulin resistance and promote the accumulation of fat. Don't disturb your fat metabolism and decrease your good cholesterol, because this has an indirect effect on losing control of managing your diabetes. Also, since diabetics have an increased risk of heart disease, all the above actions of trans fats further increase the risk of developing heart disease.

Pasta, rice and white bread

All these foods are rich in carbohydrates and quickly get digested to release lots of glucose into the blood. A study has shown that ingesting a meal consisting of a high-carb bagels resulted in significantly raising the blood glucose levels as well as decreasing the brain function in people who have type 2 diabetes. In addition, these foods are low in nutrients and have very little fiber so the overall nutritional value is almost insignificant. Food rich in fiber is important for controlling diabetes, your cholesterol levels and blood pressure and therefore the main bulk of your food should be dedicated to foods that are high in fiber.

Fruit flavored yoghurt

Simple plain yoghurt is a very healthy option for diabetics. On the contrary, yoghurt that is fruit flavored is completely different. They are often made from non-fat milk and they are loaded with carbohydrates and sugars. In fact, one serving of fruit flavored yoghurt has about 47 grams of carbohydrates in the form of sugar. Instead of choosing yogurt that is flavored and rich in sugars, opt for simple whole milk yoghurt that is free of sugar and helpful for your gut health as well as helpful to lose weight.

There are also some fruits to avoid overeating if you are diabetic.

Grapes

A single grape contains 1 gram of carbohydrates that means if you eat 30 grapes, you have easily eaten 30g of carbs. And you can eat the same number of berries or strawberries while having significantly less amount of carbohydrates.

Cherries

They are super delicious that is why it is hard to stop eating them once you have started, however, they are very rich in sugars and can cause your blood sugar to spike quickly.

Pineapple

When fresh and ripe, they can have a very high glycemic index. If you must eat pineapples try to have a small serving of about half a cup and eat it with food that is low-fat, for example, Greek yoghurt. Don't eat canned pineapple as they are sweetened with unhealthy sugars.

Mango

These are super delicious foods, however one single mango has about 30 grams of carbohydrates and about 25 grams of sugars. A riper and softer mango will have a higher glycemic index, while mango that is firm will have a lower glycemic index relatively.

Banana

It is one of those too sweet, yet very delicious foods. A medium sized banana has about the same grams of carbohydrates that is double of any other fruit.

If you must have a banana try to have half a serving and refrigerate the rest of it for another time.

Dried fruits seem harmless, especially when you add them to your food, however, two tablespoons of dried raisins have a similar amount of carbohydrates as just one cup of blueberries or another small piece of another fruit. That is because the water content has dried out and their sugars have been greatly concentrated. Remove dried fruits from your diet and add fresh ones to your diet instead.

Diabetic Plate Recipes

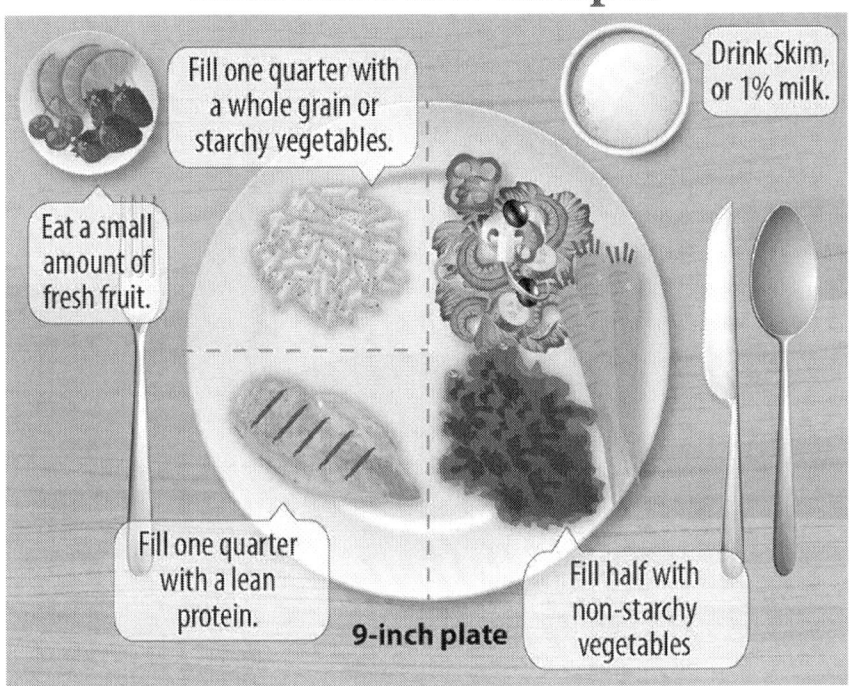

Chicken and Turkey Recipes

Pumpkin, Bean, and Chicken Enchiladas

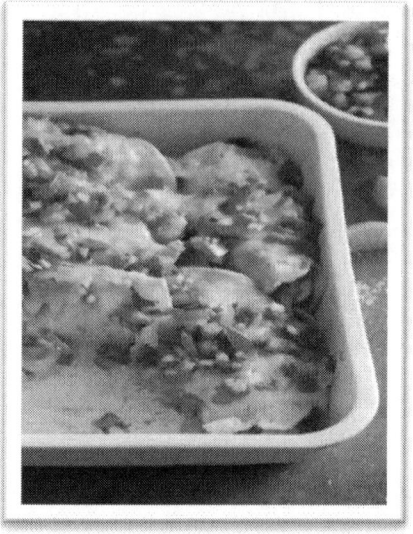

Prep time: 35 minutes	Cook time: 25 minutes	Servings: 4

Ingredients

- Olive oil – 2 tsps.
- Chopped onion – ½ cup
- Jalapeno – 1, seeded and chopped
- Pumpkin – 1 (15 oz.) can
- Water – 1 ½ cups, more if needed
- Chili powder – 1 tsp.
- Salt – ½ tsp.

- Ground cumin – ½ tsp.
- Canned no-salt-added red kidney beans – 1 cup, rinsed and drained
- Shredded cooked chicken breast – 1 ½ cups
- Shredded part-skim mozzarella cheese – ½ cup
- Whole wheat tortillas – 8 (6-inch), softened
- Salsa and lime wedges

Method

1. Lightly coat a 2-qt. rectangular baking dish with cooking spray and preheat the oven to 400F.
2. In a saucepan, heat oil over medium heat. Add jalapeno and onion and stir-fry until onion is tender, for about 5 minutes. Stir in cumin, salt, chili powder, 1 ½ cups water and pumpkin and heat through. Add more water if needed.
3. Place beans in a bowl and mash slightly with a fork. Stir in ¼ cup of the cheese, the chicken, and half of the pumpkin mixture.
4. Spoon 1/3 cup bean mixture onto each tortilla. Roll up tortillas. Place in the baking dish (seam sides down). Pour remaining pumpkin mixture over enchiladas.
5. Bake, covered, for 15 minutes. Sprinkle with remaining ¼-cup cheese. Bake, uncovered until heated through, for about 10 minutes more.
6. Serve with salsa and lime wedges.

Nutritional Facts Per Serving (2 enchiladas each)

- Calories: 357
- Fat: 8g

- Carb: 44g
- Protein: 28g

Mu Shu Chicken

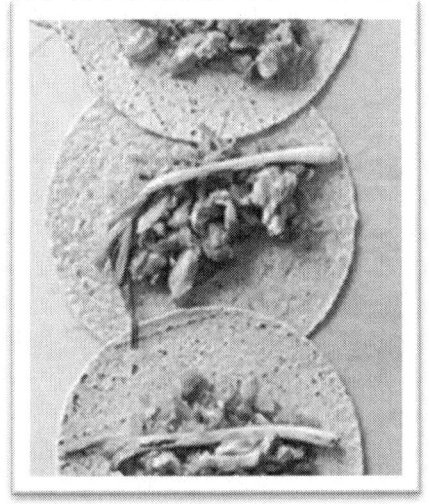

| Prep time: 20 minutes | Cook time: 6 hours | Servings: 6 |

Ingredients

- Hoisin sauce – ½ cup
- Water – 2 Tbsp.
- Toasted sesame oil - 4 tsp.
- Cornstarch – 1 Tbsp.
- Reduced-sodium soy sauce – 1 Tbsp.
- Garlic – 3 cloves, minced
- Shredded cabbage with carrots – 1 (16-oz.) pkg. (coleslaw mix)
- Coarsely shredded carrots – 1 cup

- o   Skinless, boneless chicken thighs – 12 oz.
- o   Whole wheat flour tortillas – 6 (8-inch)
- o   Green onions

Method

1. Combine the first six ingredients in a bowl (through garlic).
2. In a slow cooker, combine shredded carrots and coleslaw mix.
3. Cut chicken into 1/8 inch slices, cut each slice in half lengthwise. Place chicken on top of the cabbage mix. Drizzle with ¼ cup of the hoisin mixture.
4. Heat tortillas according to package directions. Fill tortillas with chicken mixture.
5. Top with green onions and serve.

Nutritional Facts Per Serving

- o   Calories: 269
- o   Fat: 8g
- o   Carb: 34g
- o   Protein: 16g

Stove-Top Chicken, Macaroni, and Cheese

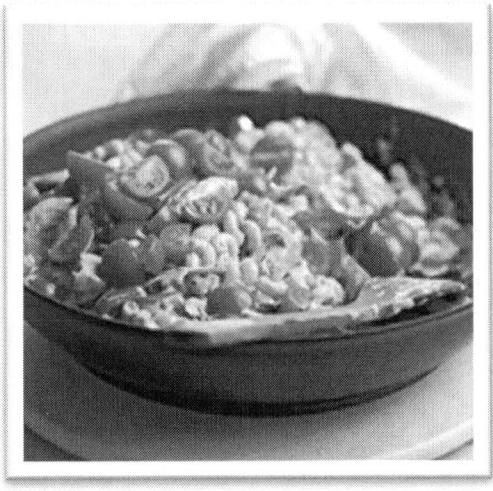

| Prep time: 10 minutes | Cook time: 30 minutes | Servings: 5 |

Ingredients

- Dried multigrain or elbow macaroni – 1 ½ cups
- Skinless, boneless chicken breast halves – 12 oz. cut into 1-inch pieces
- Chopped onion – ¼ cup
- Light semisoft cheese with garlic and fine herbs – 1 (6.5 oz.) pkg.
- Fat-free milk – 1 2/3 cups
- All-purpose flour – 1 Tbsp.
- Shredded reduced-fat cheddar cheese – ¾ cup
- Fresh baby spinach – 2 cups

- Cherry tomatoes – 1 cup, quartered

Method

1. Cook macaroni according to package directions. Drain.
2. Meanwhile, coat a skillet with cooking spray. Heat skillet over medium high heat.
3. Add onion and chicken until chicken is no longer pink, about 4 to 6 minutes. Stirring frequently. Remove from heat and stir in semisoft cheese until melted.
4. In a bowl, whisk together flour and milk until smooth. Gradually stir milk mixture into chicken mixture. Cook and stir until bubbly and thickened. Lower heat and gradually add cheddar cheese. Stirring until melted.
5. Add cooked macaroni, cook and stir for 1 to 2 minutes or until heated through.
6. Stir in spinach. Top with cherry tomatoes and serve.

Nutritional Facts Per Serving

- Calories: 369
- Fat: 12g
- Carb: 33g
- Protein: 33g

Chicken Sausage Omelets with Spinach

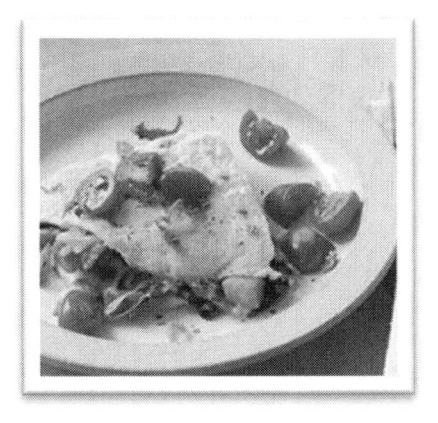

| Prep time: 20 minutes | Cook time: 10 minutes | Servings: 2 |

Ingredients

- Fresh spinach – 2 cups
- Frozen fully cooked chicken and maple breakfast sausage links – ½ of a 7-oz. pkg. thawed and chopped
- Eggs – 3, lightly beaten
- Water – 2 Tbsp.
- Shredded part-skim mozzarella cheese – ¼ cup
- Green onions – 2, green tops only, thinly sliced
- Grape tomatoes – ½ cup, quartered
- Fresh basil leaves – ¼ cup, thinly sliced

Method

1. Coat a skillet with nonstick cooking spray. Heat over medium heat.
2. Add sausage and spinach. Cook until sausage is heated. Remove from the skillet.
3. In a bowl, whisk together the water and eggs. Add egg mixture to skillet and cook until egg is set and shiny.
4. Spoon spinach and sausage mixture over half of the omelet. Sprinkle with cheese and green onions. Fold the opposite side of omelet over sausage mixture.
5. Cook for 1 minute or until filling is heated and cheese is melted.
6. Transfer to a plate and cut in half. Transfer half of the omelet to a second plate.
7. Top with tomatoes and basil and serve.

Nutritional Facts Per Serving

- Calories: 252
- Fat: 16g
- Carb: 5g
- Protein: 21g

Chicken-Broccoli Salad with Buttermilk Dressing

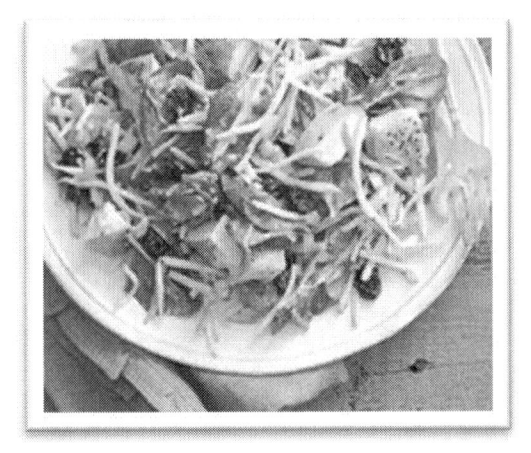

| Prep time: 20 minutes | Cook time: 0 minutes | Servings: 4 |

Ingredients

- Packaged shredded broccoli slaw mix – 3 cups
- Coarsely chopped cooked chicken breast – 2 cups
- Dried cherries – ½ cup
- Sliced celery – 1/3 cup
- Chopped red onion – ¼ cup
- Buttermilk – 1/3 cup
- Light mayonnaise – 1/3 cup
- Honey – 1 Tbsp.
- Cider vinegar – 1 Tbsp.
- Dry mustard – 1 tsp.

- Salt – ½ tsp.
- Black pepper – 1/8 tsp.
- Fresh baby spinach – 4 cups

Method

1. Combine the first five ingredients in a bowl (through onion). In a small bowl, whisk together the next seven ingredients (through pepper). Pour buttermilk mixture over broccoli mixture. Toss to gently mix.
2. Cover and chill for 2 hours to 24 hours.
3. Add baby spinach and serve.

Nutritional Facts Per Serving

- Calories: 278
- Fat: 7g
- Carb: 29g
- Protein: 26g

Country-Style Wedge Salad with Turkey

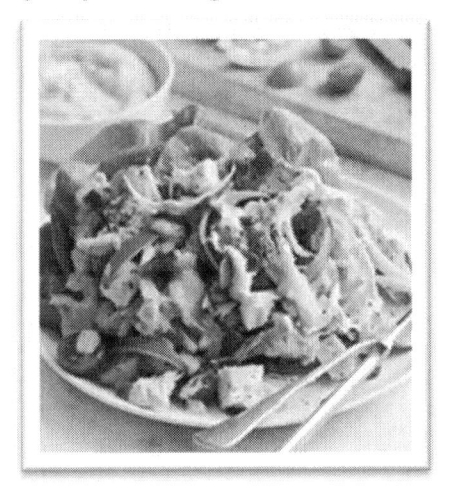

| Prep time: 10 minutes | Cook time: 0 minutes | Servings: 4 |

Ingredients

- Bibb or butterhead lettuce – 1 head, quartered
- Buttermilk-Avocado dressing – 1 recipe (see below)
- Shredded cooked turkey breast – 2 cups
- Halved grape or cherry tomatoes – 1 cup
- Hard-cooked eggs – 2, chopped
- Low-sodium, less-fat bacon – 4 slices, crisp-cooked, and crumbled
- Finely chopped red onion – ¼ cup
- Cracked black pepper

Method

1. Arrange one lettuce quarter on each plate. Drizzle half of the dressing over wedges. Top with turkey, eggs, and tomatoes. Drizzle with the remaining dressing. Sprinkle with onion, bacon and pepper.
2. To make the buttermilk-avocado dressing: in a blender, combine ¾ cup buttermilk, ½ avocado, 1 tbsp. parsley, ¼ tsp. each salt, onion powder, dry mustard, and black pepper, and 1 garlic clove, minced. Cover and blend until smooth.

Nutritional Facts Per Serving

- Calories: 228
- Fat: 9g
- Carb: 8g
- Protein: 29g

Turkey Kabob Pitas

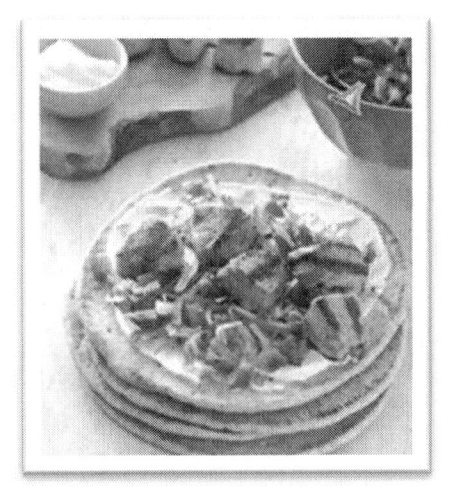

| Prep time: 25 minutes | Cook time: 15 minutes | Servings: 4 |

Ingredients

- Whole cumin seeds – 1 tsp. lightly crushed
- Shredded cucumber – 1 cup
- Seeded and chopped Roma tomato – 1/3 cup
- Slivered red onion – ¼ cup
- Shredded radishes – ¼ cup
- Snipped fresh cilantro – ¼ cup
- Black pepper – ¼ tsp.
- Turkey breast - 1 lb. cut into thin strips
- Curry blend – 1 recipe

- Plain fat-free Greek yogurt – ¼ cup
- Whole wheat pita bread rounds – 4 (6-inch)

Method

1. Soak wooden skewers in water for 30 minutes. Toast the cumin seeds for 1 minute and transfer to a bowl. Add the next six ingredients to the bowl (through pepper). Mix.
2. In another bowl, combine curry blend and turkey. Stir to coat. Thread turkey onto skewers.
3. Grill kabobs, uncovered for 6 to 8 minutes or until turkey is no longer pink. Turning kabobs occasionally.
4. Remove turkey from skewers. Spread Greek yogurt on pita breads. Spoon cucumber mixture over yogurt. Top with grilled turkey.
5. Serve.

To make the curry blend

1. In a bowl, combine 2 tsp. olive oil, 1 tsp. curry powder, ½ tsp, each ground turmeric, ground cumin, and ground coriander, ¼ tsp. ground ginger, and 1/8 tsp. salt and cayenne pepper.

Nutritional Facts Per Serving

- Calories: 343
- Fat: 6g

- Carb: 40g
- Protein: 35g

Beef and Lamb Recipes

Spicy Beef Sloppy Joes

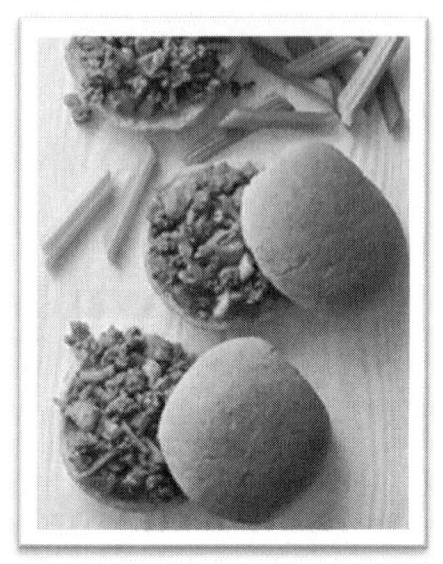

| Prep time: 20 minutes | Cook time: 8 hours | Servings: 12 |

Ingredients

- Lean ground beef – 2 lb.
- Lower-sodium salsa – 2 ½ cups
- Coarsely chopped fresh mushrooms – 3 cups
- Shredded carrots – 1 ¼ cups
- Finely chopped red and green sweet peppers – 1 ¼ cups
- No-salt added tomato paste – ½ (6-oz.) can
- Garlic – 4 cloves, minced

- Dried basil – 1 tsp. crushed
- Salt – ¾ tsp.
- Dried oregano – ½ tsp. crushed
- Cayenne pepper – ¼ tsp.
- Whole wheat hamburger buns – 12, split and toasted

Method
1. Cook ground beef in a skillet until browned. Drain off fat.
2. In a slow cooker, add the meat and combine the next 10 ingredients (through cayenne pepper).
3. Cover and cook on low for 8 to 10 hours or on high for 4 to 5 hours.
4. Spoon ½-cup of the meat mixture onto each bun.
5. Serve.

Nutritional Facts Per Serving
- Calories: 278
- Fat: 8g
- Carb: 29g
- Protein: 20g

Roasted Steak and Tomato Salad

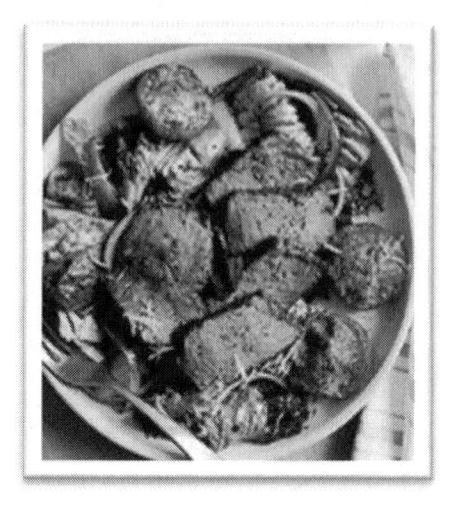

| Prep time: 20 minutes | Cook time: 20 minutes | Servings: 4 |

Ingredients

- Beef tenderloin steaks – 2 (8 oz.), trimmed
- Cracked black pepper – 1 tsp.
- Kosher salt – ¼ tsp.
- Small tomatoes – 6, halved
- Olive oil – 2 tsps.
- Shredded Parmesan cheese – ¼ cup
- Dried oregano – ½ tsp. crushed
- Torn romaine lettuce – 8 cups
- Artichoke hearts – 1 (14-oz.) can, drained and quartered
- Red onion slivers – 1/3 cup

- Balsamic vinegar – 3 Tbsp.
- Olive oil – 1 Tbsp.

Method

1. Preheat the oven to 400F.
2. Season the meat with salt and pepper and rub. Let stand for 20 minutes at room temperature.
3. Arrange tomato halves on a baking sheet (cut side down).
4. Heat 2 tsps. oil in a skillet. Add meat and cook until well browned on all sides, about 8 minutes. Transfer meat to other side of baking sheet.
5. Roast for 8 to 10 minutes for medium (145F). Remove meat from oven. Cover with foil and let stand. Move oven rack for broiling.
6. Turn oven to broil. Turn tomatoes cut sides up. Combine oregano and Parmesan. Sprinkle over tomatoes. Broil 4 to 5 inches from heat for about 2 minutes, or until cheese is melted and golden.
7. In a bowl, combine onion, artichoke hearts, and lettuce. Drizzle with vinegar and 1 tbsp. oil. Toss to coat.
8. Arrange on plates. Slice steak and arrange over lettuce with tomato halves.

Nutritional Facts Per Serving

- Calories: 299
- Fat: 14g
- Carb: 16g
- Protein: 29g

Lamb Fatteh with Asparagus

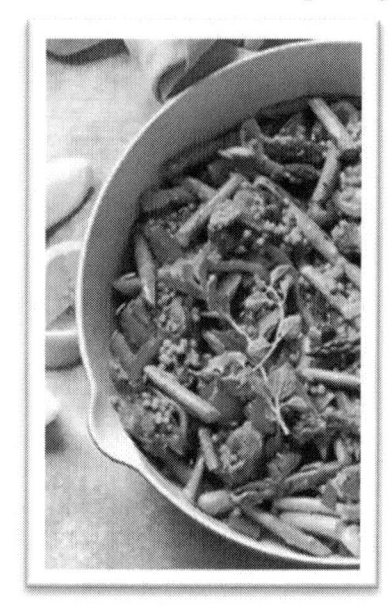

Prep time: 10 minutes	Cook time: 20 minutes	Servings: 4

Ingredients

- Olive oil – 1 Tbsp.
- Medium onion – 1, sliced
- Garlic – 4 cloves, minced
- Boneless lamb leg – 12 oz. cut into smaller pieces
- 50% less sodium beef broth – 1 (14.5 oz.) can
- Whole wheat pearl couscous - 1 cup
- Dried oregano – ½ tsp. crushed
- Ground cumin – ½ tsp.

- Salt – ¼ tsp.
- Black pepper – ¼ tsp.
- Thin asparagus spears – 1 lb. sliced into 2-inch pieces
- Chopped red sweet pepper – ¾ cup
- Snipped fresh oregano and lemon wedges

Method

1. Heat oil in a skillet. Add onion and cook for 3 minutes.
2. Add garlic and cook for 1 minute.
3. Add lamb and cook until browned on all sides, about 3 to 5 minutes.
4. Stir in the next six ingredients (through black pepper). Bring to a boil. Lower heat and simmer, covered, for 10 minutes. Stirring occasionally.
5. Stir in sweet pepper and asparagus. Cover and simmer until vegetables are crisp-tender, about 3 to 5 minutes.
6. Fluff lamb mixture lightly with a fork. Top with fresh oregano.
7. Serve with lemon wedges.

Nutritional Facts Per Serving

- Calories: 334
- Fat: 9g
- Carb: 39g
- Protein: 26g

Beef Goulash Soup

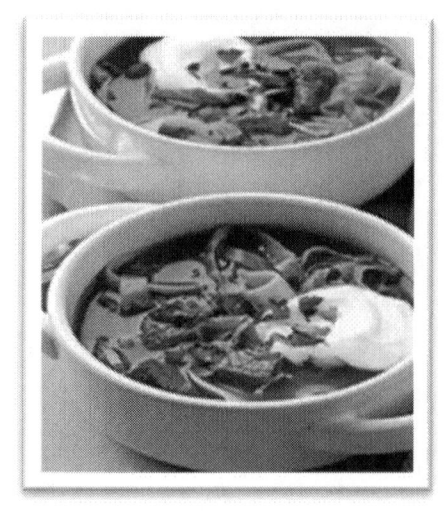

| Prep time: 30 minutes | Cook time: 20 minutes | Servings: 4 |

Ingredients

- Boneless beef top sirloin steak – 6 oz.
- Olive oil – 1 tsp.
- Chopped onion – ½ cup
- Water – 2 cups
- Beef broth – 1 (14.5 oz.) can
- No-salt-added diced tomatoes – 1 (14.5 oz.) can, undrained
- Thinly sliced carrot – ½ cup
- Unsweetened cocoa powder – 1 tsp.
- Garlic – 1 clove, minced

- o   Thinly sliced cabbage – 1 cup
- o   Dried wide noodles – ½ cup
- o   Paprika – 2 tsps.
- o   Light sour cream – ¼ cup
- o   Snipped fresh parsley

Method

1. Cut meat into ½-inch cubes. In a saucepan, cook and stir meat in hot oil until browned, for about 6 minutes. Add onion, cook and stir until onion softens, about 3 minutes.
2. Stir in the next six ingredients (through garlic). Bring to a boil. Reduce heat. Simmer, uncovered, for about 15 minutes or until meat is tender.
3. Stir in paprika, noodles, and cabbage. Simmer, uncovered, until noodles are tender but still firm, for about 5 to 7 minutes. Remove from heat.
4. Top each serving with sour cream.
5. Sprinkle with parsley and additional paprika.
6. Serve.

Nutritional Facts Per Serving

- o   Calories: 188
- o   Fat: 7g
- o   Carb: 16g
- o   Protein: 14g

Beef-Vegetable Ragout

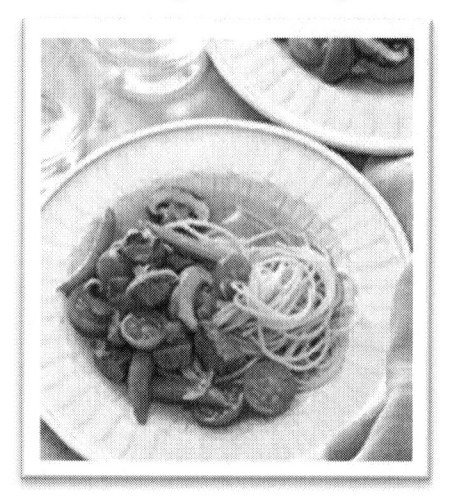

Prep time: 30 minutes	Cook time: 8 hours	Servings: 8

Ingredients

- Beef chuck roast – 1 ½ lb.
- Sliced fresh button or cremini mushrooms – 3 cups
- Chopped onion – 1 cup
- Garlic – 4 cloves, minced
- Salt – ½ tsp.
- Black pepper – ½ tsp.
- Quick-cooking tapioca -1/4 cup, crushed
- 50% less-sodium beef broth – 2 (14.5 oz.) cans
- Dry sherry – ½ cup
- Sugar snap pea pods – 4 cups

- o Cherry tomatoes – 2 cups, halved
- o Hot cooked multigrain noodles – 4 cups

Method

1. Cut meat into ¾-inch pieces.
2. Coat a skillet with cooking spray. Cook meat, half at a time, in the hot skillet until browned.
3. Combine the next five ingredients (through pepper) in a slow cooker. Sprinkle with tapioca. Add meat and pour in broth and dry sherry.
4. Cover and cook on low for 8 to 10 hours or high for 4 to 5 hours.
5. If slow cooker is on low, turn to high. Stir in sugar snap peas. Cover and cook for 5 minutes.
6. Stir in cherry tomatoes. Serve meat mixture over hot cooked noodles.

Nutritional Facts Per Serving

- o Calories: 208
- o Fat: 4g
- o Carb: 19g
- o Protein: 24g

Greek Flat Iron Steaks

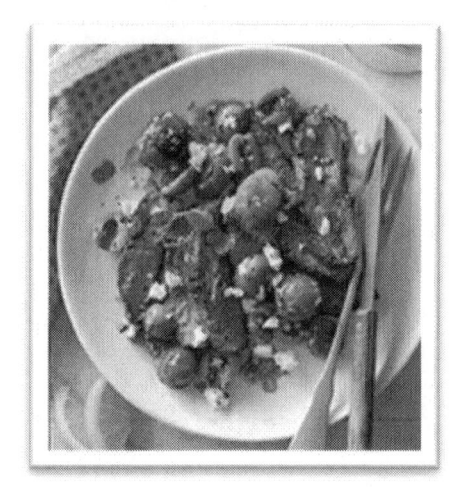

| Prep time: 10 minutes | Cook time: 15 minutes | Servings: 4 |

Ingredients

- Lemon – 1
- Boneless beef shoulder top blade steaks (flat iron) – 2 (6 to 8 oz.)
- Salt – ¼ tsp.
- Black pepper – ¼ tsp.
- Dried rosemary – 1 tsp. crushed
- Olive oil – 4 tsp.
- Grape tomatoes – 2 cups, halved
- Garlic – 2 cloves, minced
- Pitted green olives – 1/3 cup, halved

- Crumbled feta cheese – ¼ cup
- Lemon wedges

Method

1. Remove 1 tsp. zest from the lemon. Set zest aside. Cut steaks in half and season with salt and pepper. Sprinkle rosemary on both sides of the steaks.
2. Heat 2 tsps. oil in a skillet. Add steaks and cook until medium rare, about 8 to 10 minutes. Turning once. Remove and set aside.
3. Add remaining 2 tsps. oil to the skillet. Add garlic and tomatoes. Cook until tomatoes are soft and burst, for about 3 minutes. Remove from heat. Stir in the lemon zest and olives.
4. Serve steaks with tomato relish.
5. Sprinkle with cheese and serve with the reserved lemon wedges.

Nutritional Facts Per Serving

- Calories: 223
- Fat: 14g
- Carb: 6g
- Protein: 20g

Spiced Burgers with Cilantro Cucumber Sauce

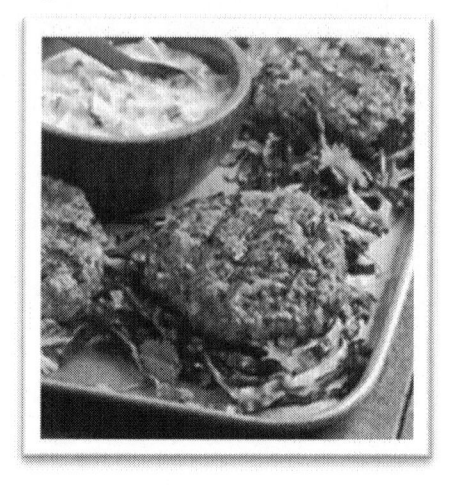

Prep time: 25 minutes	Cook time: 15 minutes	Servings: 4

Ingredients

- Plain fat-free Greek yogurt – 1 (5.3 to 6 oz.) container
- Finely chopped cucumber – 2/3 cup
- Snipped fresh cilantro – ¼ cup
- Garlic – 2 cloves, minced
- Salt – 1/8 tsp.
- Black pepper – 1/8 tsp.
- Canned garbanzo beans – ½ cup, rinsed and drained
- Lean ground beef – 1 lb.
- Finely chopped red onion – ¼ cup
- Chopped jalapeno pepper – 2 Tbsps.

- Salt – ½ tsp.
- Ground cumin – ¼ tsp.
- Ground coriander – ¼ tsp.
- Cinnamon – 1/8 tsp.
- Black pepper – 1/8 tsp.
- Radicchio – 1 head, shredded

Method

1. To make the sauce: in a bowl, stir together the first six ingredients (through black pepper). Cover and keep in the refrigerator.
2. In a bowl, mash garbanzo beans with a fork. Add the next eight ingredients (through black pepper), mix well. Form meat mixture into four ¾ inch thick patties.
3. Grill burgers, covered, over medium 14 to 18 minutes or until done (160F). Turning once.
4. Toss radicchio with additional fresh cilantro leaves.
5. Serve burgers on radicchio, top with sauce.

Nutritional Facts Per Serving

- Calories: 258
- Fat: 12g
- Carb: 8g
- Protein: 29g

Fish and Seafood Recipes

Caribbean Fish with Mango-Orange Relish

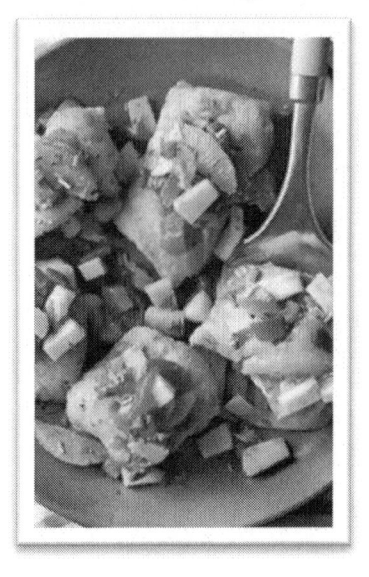

Prep time: 25 minutes	Cook time: 15 minutes	Servings: 6

Ingredients

- Fresh or frozen skinless barramundi, sea bass, or other whitefish fillets – 2 ½ lb.
- Navel oranges – 3
- Large mango – 1, chopped
- Chopped roasted red sweet pepper – ¾ cup
- Dry white wine – 2 Tbsps.
- Snipped fresh cilantro – 1 Tbsp.
- Salt – ¼ tsp.

- Black pepper – ¼ tsp.
- All-purpose flour – 1/3 cup
- Ground cardamom – 2 tsps.
- Butter – ¼ cup
- Snipped fresh chives

Method

1. For relish, juice one of the oranges. Peel and section the remaining two oranges. Combine orange sections, orange juice and the next four ingredients (through cilantro).
2. Sprinkle fish with salt and pepper. In a dish, combine cardamom and flour. Dip fish in flour mixture, turning to coat.
3. Preheat oven to 300F. In a skillet, melt 2 tbsps. butter. Add half of the fish. Cook until fish is golden and flakes easily, about 6 to 8 minutes. Turning once.
4. Cook the remaining fish in remaining 2 Tbsps. butter. Serve with relish and sprinkle with chives.

Nutritional Facts Per Serving

- Calories: 343
- Fat: 12g
- Carb: 20g
- Protein: 37g

Lemon-Herb Roasted Salmon Sheet-Pan Dinner

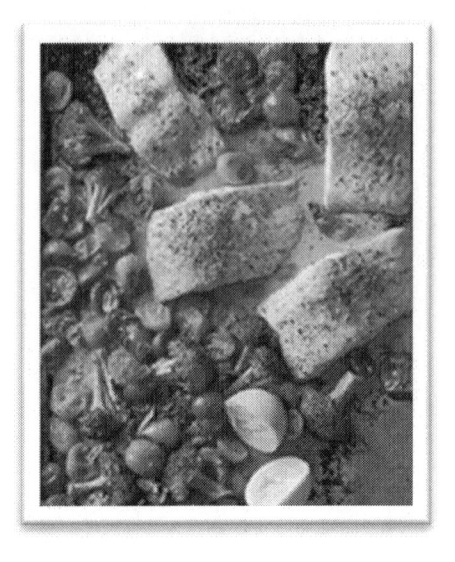

Prep time: 20 minutes	Cook time: 15 minutes	Servings: 4

Ingredients

- Fresh or frozen skinless salmon fillet – 1 (1 lb.)
- Olive oil – 2 Tbsps.
- Dried oregano – 1 ½ tsp. crushed
- Salt – ¼ tsp.
- Black pepper – 1/8 tsp.
- Grape or cherry tomatoes – 2 cups halved
- Broccoli florets – 2 cups
- Garlic – 2 cloves, minced
- Lemon – 1

- Snipped fresh basil – 2 Tbsp.
- Snipped fresh parsley – 1 Tbsp.
- Honey – 1 Tbsp.

Method

1. Thaw salmon, if frozen. Preheat oven to 400F.
2. Line a baking pan with parchment paper.
3. Rinse fish and pat dry.
4. Place salmon in the prepared pan. Drizzle with 1 tbsp. oil and sprinkle with ¾ tsp. oregano, salt and pepper.
5. In a bowl, combine garlic, broccoli, tomatoes, and remaining 1 tbsp. oil and ¾ tsp. oregano. Sprinkle lightly with more salt and pepper. Toss to coat.
6. Place in the pan with salmon. Roast until salmon flakes, about 15 to 18 minutes.
7. Meanwhile, remove 1 tsp. zest and squeeze 3 tbsps. juice from lemon. In a small bowl, combine lemon juice and zest and remaining ingredients.
8. Spoon over salmon and vegetables before serving.

Nutritional Facts Per Serving

- Calories: 276
- Fat: 14g
- Carb: 13g
- Protein: 25g

Shrimp and Chicken Dumpling Soup

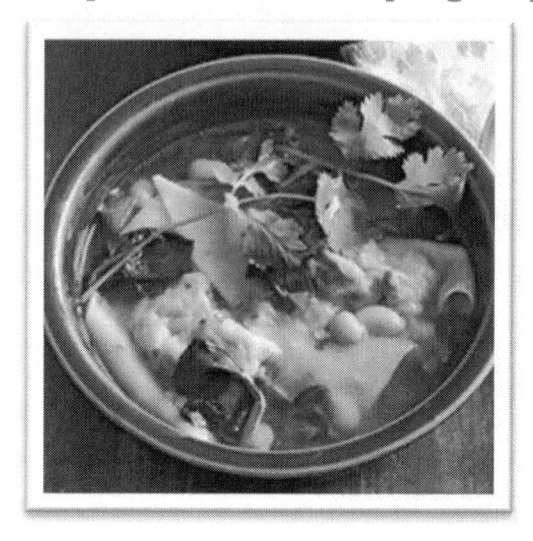

| Prep time: 10 minutes | Cook time: 5 minutes | Servings: 6 |

Ingredients

- Frozen peeled, cooked shrimp – 1 (6 oz.) pkg. thawed and finely chopped
- Chopped cooked chicken – ½ cup
- Chopped fresh mushrooms – ½ cup
- Reduced-sodium soy sauce – 2 Tbsps.
- Sliced green onions – ½ cup
- Snipped fresh cilantro – ¼ cup
- Wonton wrappers – 24
- Low-sodium chicken broth – 6 cups

- Chopped red sweet pepper – ¾ cup
- Frozen edamame – ½ cup
- Salt – ¼ tsp.
- Fresh baby spinach – 2 cups
- Toasted sesame oil – 2 tsps.

Method

1. For filling, combine the first four ingredients (through soy sauce), ¼ cup of the green onions, and 2 tsps. cilantro.
2. Working with two wonton wrappers at a time, top each with a rounded tsp. of the filling. Brush edges of the wrappers with water. Fold and seal edges. Repeat with the remaining.
3. In a saucepan, combine the next four ingredients (through salt) and the remaining green onions and cilantro.
4. Bring to a boil. Slowly add wontons to boiling broth mixture. Boil gently until tender, about 2 to 3 minutes. Stirring occasionally.
5. Stir in sesame oil and spinach.
6. Top with additional snipped fresh cilantro and serve.

Nutritional Facts Per Serving

- Calories: 189
- Fat: 3g
- Carb: 24g
- Protein: 17g

Cod with Eggplant Peperonata

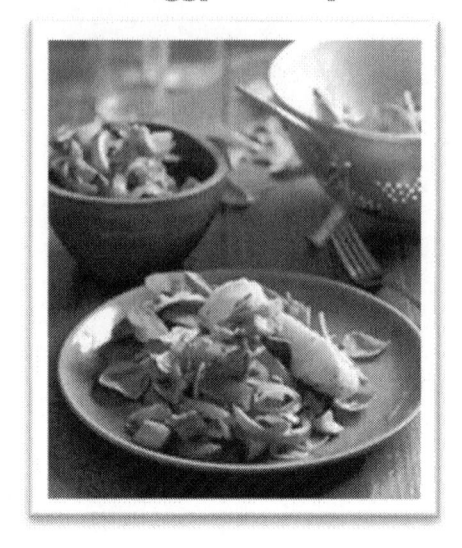

| Prep time: 10 minutes | Cook time: 25 minutes | Servings: 4 |

Ingredients

- Fresh or frozen cod fillets – 4 (4-oz.)
- Medium sweet onion – ½, thinly sliced
- Olive oil – 1 Tbsp.
- Small eggplant – 1, cut into 1-inch pieces
- Yellow or red sweet pepper – 1 large, thinly sliced
- Garlic – 4 cloves, minced
- Snipped fresh rosemary – 1 tsp.
- Salt – ½ tsp.
- Black pepper – ¼ tsp.

- Fresh spinach – 4 cups

Method

1. Thaw fish, if frozen. Rinse fish, pat dry with paper towels.
2. For eggplant peperonata, in a skillet, cook onion in hot oil for 5 minutes. Stirring occasionally.
3. Add the next four ingredients (through rosemary), and ¼ tsp. salt. Cook until vegetables are very tender, about 10 to 12 minutes. Stirring occasionally. Remove peperonata from skillet and keep warm.
4. Add 1-inch of water to the same skillet. Place a steamer basket in the skillet and bring the water to boil. Sprinkle cod with the remaining ¼ tsp. salt and the black pepper.
5. Add fish to the steamer basket. Cover and reduce heat to medium. Steam just until fish flakes, about 6 to 8 minutes.
6. Top spinach with fish and eggplant peperonata.

Nutritional Facts Per Serving

- Calories: 189
- Fat: 5g
- Carb: 13g
- Protein: 23g

Parmesan-Crusted Cod with Garlicky Summer Squash

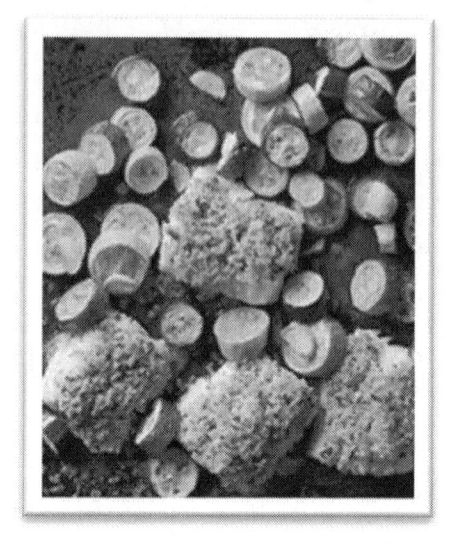

| Prep time: 20 minutes | Cook time: 20 minutes | Servings: 4 |

Ingredients

- Fresh or frozen skinless cod fillets – 4 (5 to 6 oz.) fillets
- Small zucchini or yellow summer squash – 4, cut into ¾ inch pieces
- Garlic – 2 cloves, minced
- Olive oil – ¼ cup
- Salt – ¼ tsp.
- Black pepper – 1/8 tsp.
- Panko breadcrumbs – ¼ cup
- Grated Parmesan cheese – ¼ cup

- o   Snipped fresh parsley – 2 Tbsp.

Method

1. Preheat the oven to 350F. in a baking pan, combine garlic and squash.
2. Drizzle with 2 tbsp. oil. Rinse and pat dry fish. Place in pan with squash. Sprinkle fish and squash with 1/8 tsp. of the salt and pepper.
3. In a bowl, combine parsley, cheese, panko, and remaining 1/8 tsp. salt. Drizzle with the remaining 2 tbsp. oil and toss to coat.
4. Sprinkle eon top of the fish. Press lightly.
5. Bake for about 20 minutes or until fish flakes.
6. Sprinkle with additional parsley.
7. Serve.

Nutritional Facts Per Serving

- o   Calories: 297
- o   Fat: 16g
- o   Carb: 8g
- o   Protein: 29g

Fried Cauliflower Rice with Shrimp

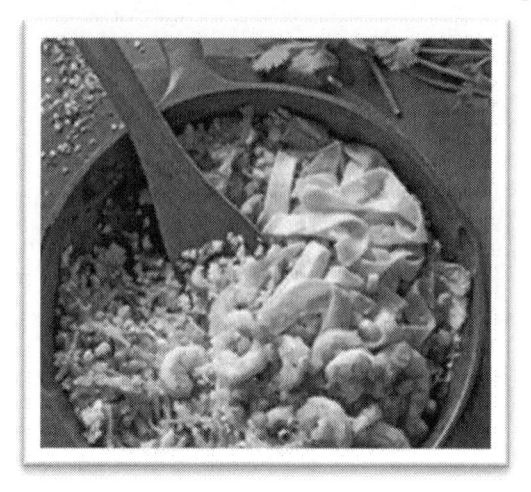

| Prep time: 10 minutes | Cook time: 10 minutes | Servings: 4 |

Ingredients

- Fresh or frozen medium shrimp – 8 oz. peeled and deveined
- Cauliflower – 1 (2 lb.) head, cut into florets
- Toasted sesame oil – 1 tsp.
- Eggs – 2, lightly beaten
- Olive oil – 1 Tbsp.
- Grated fresh ginger – 4 tsp.
- Garlic – 4 cloves, minced
- Chopped napa cabbage – 2 cups
- Coarsely shredded carrots – 1 cup

- Sea salt – ½ tsp.
- Crushed red pepper – ½ tsp.
- Sliced green onions – 1/3 cup
- Snipped fresh cilantro – 2 Tbsp.
- Lime wedges

Method

1. Thaw shrimp if frozen. Rinse shrimp and pat dry.
2. Pulse cauliflower in a food processor until rice size.
3. In a skillet, heat sesame oil over medium heat. Add eggs, stir gently until set. Remove eggs and cool slightly. Cut eggs into strips.
4. Heat the olive oil in the skillet over medium heat. Add garlic and ginger. Cook for 30 seconds.
5. Add carrots and cabbage and stir-fry until vegetables start to soften, about 2 minutes.
6. Add crushed red pepper, salt, and shrimp. Stir-fry for 2 minutes or until shrimp are opaque.
7. Add green onions, and cooked egg. Stir-fry until heated through.
8. Shrink shrimp mixture with cilantro. Serve with lemon wedges.

Nutritional Facts Per Serving

- Calories: 181
- Fat: 8g
- Carb: 14g
- Protein: 17g

Quick Scallop and Noodle Toss

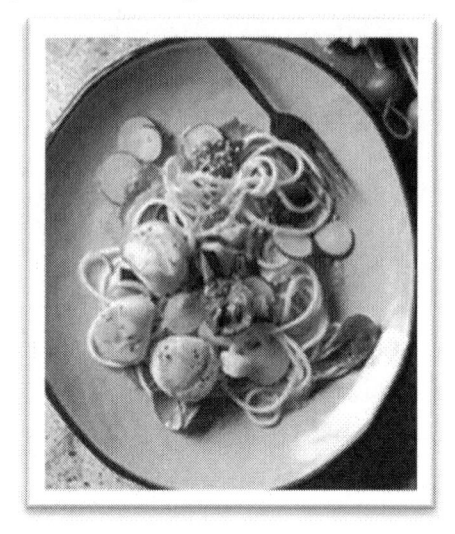

| Prep time: 5 minutes | Cook time: 10 minutes | Servings: 4 |

Ingredients

- Fresh or frozen sea scallops – 12
- Medium zucchini – 1, trimmed
- Olive oil – ½ tsp.
- Orange juice – 2 Tbsps.
- Cider vinegar – 2 Tbsps.
- Toasted sesame oil – 1 Tbsp.
- Grated fresh ginger – 1 tsp.
- Lime zest – ½ tsp.
- Sea salt – ½ tsp.

- o Fresh baby spinach – 1 ½ cups
- o Chopped cucumber – 1 cup
- o Thinly sliced radishes – 2/3 cups
- o Black pepper – ¼ tsp.
- o Olive oil – 1 Tbsp.
- o Sesame seeds – 2 Tbsps. toasted

Method

1. Thaw scallops, if frozen. Cut zucchini into long, thin noodles.
2. Heat ½ tsp. olive oil in a skillet. Add zucchini noodles and stir-fry for 1 minute or until tender. Cool.
3. Meanwhile, in a bowl, combine the next five ingredients (through lime zest) and ¼ tsp. salt. Stir in radishes, cucumber, spinach, and zucchini noodles.
4. Rinse scallops and pat dry. Sprinkle with remaining ¼ tsp. salt and pepper.
5. Heat 1 tbsp. olive oil in the same skillet. Add the scallops and cook until opaque, about 3 to 5 minutes. Turning once.
6. Serve zucchini noodle mixture with scallops and sprinkle with sesame seeds.

Nutritional Facts Per Serving

- o Calories: 227
- o Fat: 10g
- o Carb: 9g
- o Protein: 24g

Meatless/Vegan Recipes

Falafel and Vegetable Pitas

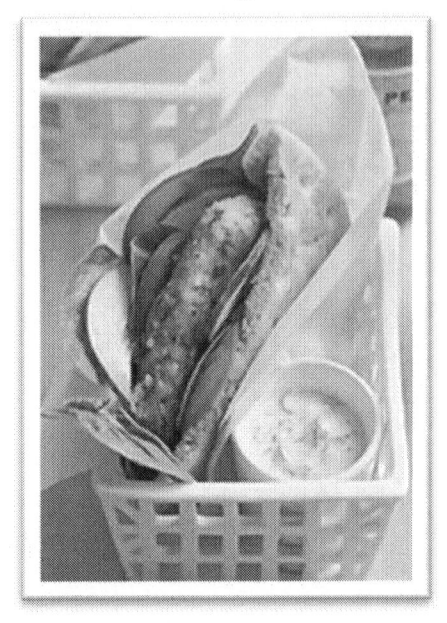

Prep time: 25 minutes	Cook time: 5 minutes	Servings: 4

Ingredients

- Lemon – 1
- Reduced-sodium garbanzo beans – 1 (15-oz.)can, rinsed and drained
- Whole-wheat flour – 2 Tbsps.
- Snipped fresh Italian parsley – 2 Tbsps.
- Garlic – 3 cloves, sliced
- Ground coriander – ½ tsp.

- Salt – ¼ tsp.
- Black pepper – ¼ tsp.
- Ground cumin – 1/8 tsp.
- Whole grain pita bread rounds – 2, halved
- Fresh spinach or watercress – ¾ cup
- Roma tomato – 8 thin slices
- Thinly sliced cucumber – ½ cup
- Yogurt sauce – 1 recipe

Method

1. Remove 2 tsps. zest and squeeze 2 tbsps. juice from lemon.
2. To make the falafel, in a food processor, combine the juice, zest, and the next eight ingredients (through cumin). Cover and process until finely chopped.
3. Shape garbanzo bean mixture into four ½-inch thick oval patties. Coat a skillet with cooking spray and heat over medium heat.
4. Add patties and cook until browned, for about 4 to 6 minutes. Turning once.
5. Open pita halves to make pockets. Fill pockets with cucumber slices, tomato slices, and spinach.
6. Add falafel and top with yogurt sauce.
7. Serve.

To make the yogurt sauce: in a bowl stir together ½ cup plain fat-free yogurt, 1/8 tsp. each of salt, and black pepper, and 2 tbsp. fresh Italian parsley.

Nutritional Facts Per Serving

- Calories: 217
- Fat: 3g
- Carb: 43g
- Protein: 11g

Chickpea Alfredo with Spring Veggies

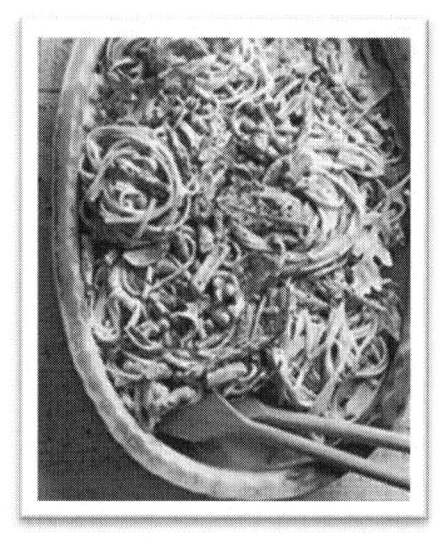

| Prep time: 10 minutes | Cook time: 25 minutes | Servings: 6 |

Ingredients

- Unsalted raw cashews – 1/3 cup
- Boiling water
- Dried whole grain or brown rice fettuccine – 12 oz.
- Chopped fresh asparagus – 1 cup
- Lightly packed fresh spinach or arugula – 2 cups
- Frozen peas – ½ cup, slightly thawed
- Water – 1 ¼ cup
- Garbanzo bean – ¼ cup, flour
- Lemon juice – 1 Tbsp.

- Olive oil – 2 tsps.
- Garlic – 2 cloves, minced
- Kosher salt and black pepper to taste
- Snipped fresh basil – 2 Tbsps.
- Shaved parmesan cheese

Method

1. In a small bowl, combine cashews and enough boiling water to cover. Let stand, covered, 20 minutes, then drain. Rinse and drain again.
2. Meanwhile, cook pasta according to package directions. Add asparagus in the last 3 minutes and add spinach and peas in the last 1 minute of cooking. Drain.
3. In a small saucepan, whisk together the flour and water until smooth. Cook and stir over medium heat until just until bubbly.
4. For sauce, in a blender, combine soaked cashews, flour mixture, and the next five ingredients (through pepper). Cover and pulse several times. Then blend until smooth. Transfer pasta mixture to a serving dish.
5. Drizzle with sauce. Toss to coat.
6. Sprinkle with more pepper and parmesan cheese.
7. Serve.

Nutritional Facts Per Serving

- Calories: 290
- Fat: 7g
- Carb: 49g
- Protein: 11g

Mediterranean Fried Quinoa

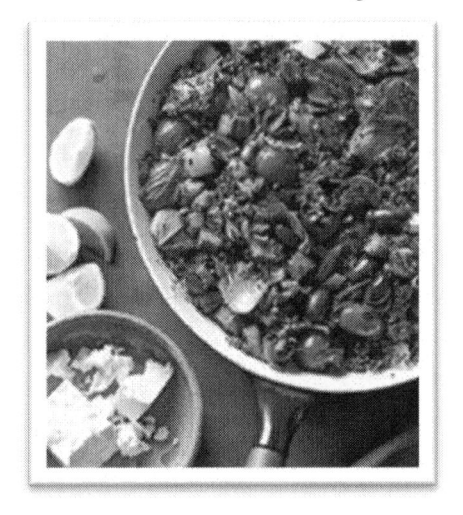

| Prep time: 10 minutes | Cook time: 25 minutes | Servings: 4 |

Ingredients

- Reduced-sodium chicken broth – 2 cups
- Red quinoa – 1 cup
- Olive oil – 1 Tbsp.
- Eggplant – 3 cups, ½ inch pieces
- Coarsely chopped onion – ¾ cup
- Garlic – 2 cloves, minced
- Black pepper – ¼ tsp.
- Grape tomatoes – 1 cup
- Fresh baby spinach – 4 cups
- Pitted Kalamata olives – ¼ cup, halved

- o   Snipped fresh oregano – 1 Tbsp.
- o   Crumbled feta cheese – ¼ cup
- o   Lemon wedges

Method

1. In a saucepan, bring broth to boiling. Add quinoa and return to boiling. Lower heat, simmer, covered, until liquid is absorbed, about 15 minutes. Remove from heat. Drain and return quinoa to saucepan. Cook and stir over low heat to dry excess moisture from quinoa.
2. Heat oil in a skillet. Add quinoa and cook until starts to brown, about 2 to 4 minutes. Add pepper, garlic, onion, and eggplant. Stir-fry for 3 minutes.
3. Add tomatoes, and stir-fry for 2 minutes or until tomatoes start to burst. Remove from heat. Add spinach, oregano, and olives. Toss.
4. Sprinkle with feta cheese and serve with lemon wedges.

Nutritional Facts Per Serving

- o   Calories: 291
- o   Fat: 10g
- o   Carb: 41g
- o   Protein: 11g

Asparagus and Greens with Farro

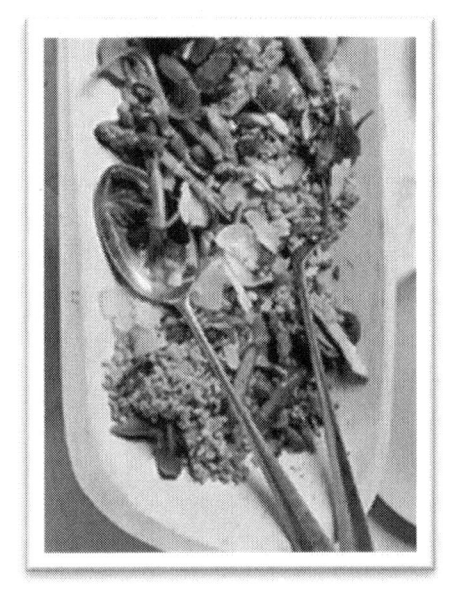

| Prep time: 10 minutes | Cook time: 30 minutes | Servings: 4 |

Ingredients

- Water – 3 cups
- Uncooked farro – 1 cup
- Thin asparagus – 1 bunch, trimmed and cut into 2-inch pieces
- Lemon juice – 3 Tbsps.
- Whole almonds – ½ cup, toasted and chopped
- Olive oil – 1 Tbsp.
- Kosher salt – ½ tsp.
- Black pepper – ¼ tsp.

- Baby spinach and/or baby kale – 3 cups
- Shaved Parmesan cheese – 1/3 cup

Method

1. In a saucepan, bring water to boil. Add farro, lower heat, simmer, covered, until just tender, about 30 minutes. Drain.
2. Meanwhile, place a steamer basket in a skillet. Add water to just below basket. Bring water to boil.
3. Add asparagus to basket. Cover, and steam until crisp-tender, about 3 minutes. Transfer to a large bowl.
4. Add farro to bowl with asparagus. Drizzle with lemon juice and stir in pepper, salt, olive oil, and almonds. Add greens and toss to combine. Top with Parmesan.

Nutritional Facts Per Serving

- Calories: 360
- Fat: 15g
- Carb: 43g
- Protein: 15g

Toasted Walnut Tempeh Tacos

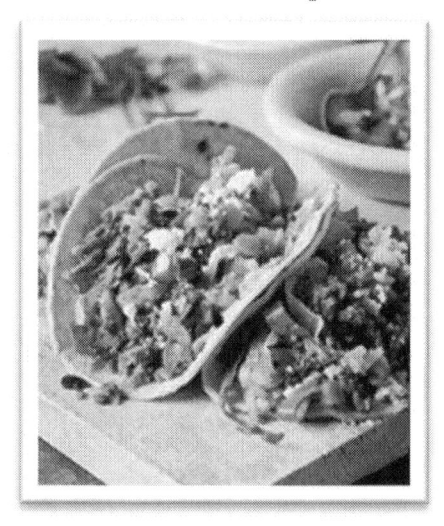

| Prep time: 5 minutes | Cook time: 15 minutes | Servings: 4 |

Ingredients

- Fresh poblano pepper – 1 medium, seeded and chopped
- Chopped onion – ½ cup
- Tempeh – 1 (8-oz.) pkg. crumbled
- Garlic – 2 cloves, minced
- Salt-free Mexican-seasoning blend – 2 tsps.
- Salt – ¼ tsp.
- Chopped walnuts – ¼ cup, toasted
- Chopped avocado – ½ cup
- Lime juice – ½ tsp.

- Salt – 1/8 tsp.
- Corn tortillas – 8 (6-inch), warmed
- Shredded romaine lettuce – 1 ½ cups
- Refrigerated fresh salsa – 1 cup
- Crumbled Cotija cheese – ¼ cup
- Chopped fresh cilantro – ½ cup

Method

1. Coat a skillet with cooking spray and heat over medium heat.
2. Add onion and pepper and cook until vegetables are crisp-tender, about 3 to 5 minutes. Stirring occasionally.
3. Add the next four ingredients (though salt). Cook until heated and tempeh is lightly browned, about 6 to 8 minutes. Stirring occasionally. Remove from heat and stir in walnuts.
4. Meanwhile, in a small bowl, mash avocado with 1/8 tsp. salt, and lime juice. Spread mashed avocado over tortillas, then top with lettuce.
5. Spoon warm tempeh mixture over lettuce. Top with cilantro, cheese, and salsa.

Nutritional Facts Per Serving

- Calories: 380
- Fat: 19g
- Carb: 37g
- Protein: 18g

Mushroom-Lentil Shepard's Pie

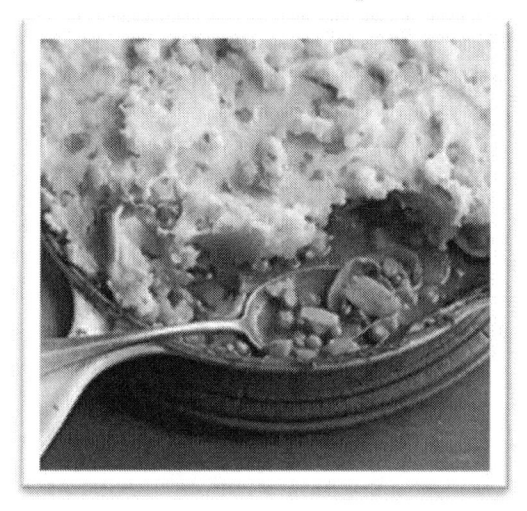

| Prep time: 10 minutes | Cook time: 50 minutes | Servings: 6 |

Ingredients

- Vegetable broth – 2 cups
- Dried brown lentils – ½ cup, rinsed and drained
- Dried rosemary – ½ tsp. crushed
- Dried thyme – ½ tsp. crushed
- Round red potatoes – 2 ½ lb. cut into 1-inch pieces
- Garlic – 2 cloves, peeled
- Butter – 5 Tbsps.
- Salt – ¾ tsp.
- Sliced fresh mushrooms – 3 cups

- Chopped onion – 1 cup
- Frozen peas and carrots – 1 ½ cups
- Reduced-sodium soy sauce – 4 tsps.
- Cornstarch - 1 Tbsp.
- Worcestershire sauce – 2 tsps.

Method

1. Bring 1 cup water to boil in a saucepan. Add lentils, rosemary, and thyme. Simmer, covered, until tender, about 30 to 40 minutes. Drain.
2. Meanwhile, preheat oven to 375F.
3. In a Dutch oven, cook potatoes, and garlic in boiling water until potatoes are tender, about 15 minutes. Drain, and reserve ½ cup cooking water. Coarsely mash potatoes. Mash in the salt and 3 tbsps. butter. Stir in enough reserved cooking water to reach desired consistency.
4. Heat 1 tbsp. butter in a skillet. Add onion and mushrooms and cook for 10 minutes. Stirring occasionally. Stir in carrots and peas.
5. In a small bowl, combine the 1 cup broth, Worcestershire sauce, soy sauce, and cornstarch. Stir into the mushroom mixture.
6. Stir-fry until thickened and bubbly. Cook and stir 1 minute more. Stir in cooked lentils.
7. Top lentil mixture with mashed potatoes, spreading to edges. Dot with remaining 1 tbsp. butter.
8. Transfer skillet to the oven and bake until potatoes start to brown, about 20 minutes.

Nutritional Facts Per Serving

- Calories: 328
- Fat: 10g
- Carb: 51g
- Protein: 11g

Sesame-Mustard Oats with Charred Green Onions

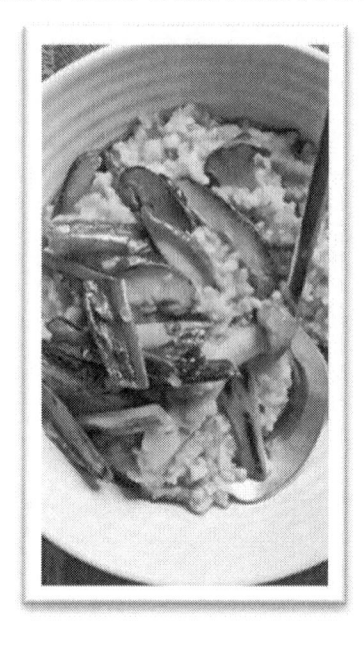

| Prep time: 15 minutes | Cook time: 30 minutes | Servings: 1 |

Ingredients

- Reduced-sodium chicken broth – 1 cup
- Steel-cut oats – ½ cup
- Toasted sesame oil – 2 tsps.
- Assorted fresh mushrooms – 1 cup, sliced
- Minced fresh ginger – 1 tsp.
- Green onions – 2, cut into 1-inch pieces
- Reduced-sodium soy sauce – 1 tsp.
- Crushed red pepper

Method

1. Bring broth to a boil in a saucepan. Stir in oats. Reduce heat to medium-low. Cook, uncovered, until oats are tender, and mixture is thickened and creamy, about 25 to 30 minutes. Stirring occasionally.
2. Meanwhile, heat 1 tsp. oil in a skillet. Add ginger and mushrooms and cook until tender, about 3 to 4 minutes. Transfer to a bowl.
3. Add remaining oil to skillet. Increase heat to medium-high. Add green onions and cook until charred, about 2 minutes. Remove from heat.
4. Stir mushrooms into oats.
5. Top with crushed red pepper, green onions, and soy sauce.
6. Serve.

Nutritional Facts Per Serving

- Calories: 474
- Fat: 15g
- Carb: 65g
- Protein: 21g

Desserts

Frozen Yogurt Bark

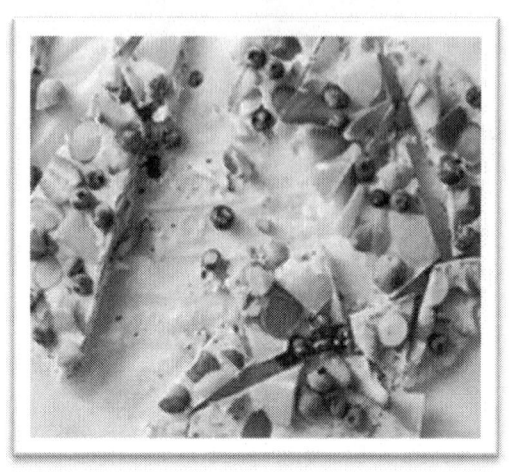

| Prep time: 15 minutes | Freeze time: 2 hours | Servings: 24 |

Ingredients

- Plain Whole-milk Greek yogurt – 1 (32-oz.) carton
- Honey – ¼ cup
- Vanilla extract – 2 tsp.
- Filling – 1 cup (chopped berries, nuts, dark chocolate)
- Toppers – 2 cups (cacao nibs, seeds, nuts, fruit, toasted raw chip coconut)

Method

1. Line two large baking sheet with parchment paper. In a bowl, combine vanilla, honey, and yogurt. Stir in fillings.

2. Divide yogurt mixture between prepared baking sheets, spreading into rectangles. Sprinkle with toppers.
3. Freeze 2 to 4 hours or until firm. Break bark into 24 irregular pieces.
4. Serve.

Nutritional Facts Per Serving

- Calories: 117
- Fat: 7g
- Carb: 9g
- Protein: 5g

Sweet Ricotta and Strawberry Parfaits

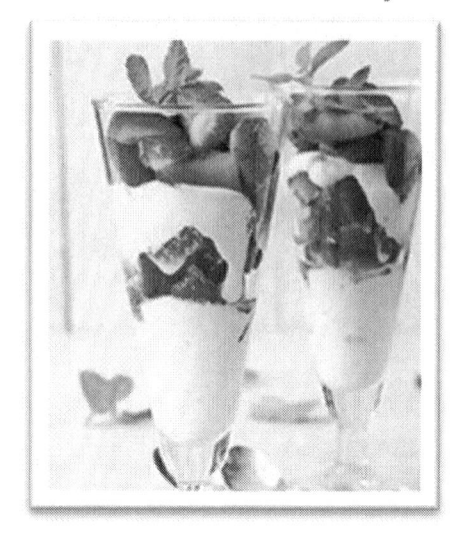

Prep time: 10 minutes	Cook time: 0 minutes	Servings: 6

Ingredients

- Fresh strawberries – 1 lb. quartered
- Snipped fresh mint – 1 Tbsp.
- Sugar – 1 tsp.
- Part-skim ricotta cheese – 1 (15-oz.) carton
- Honey – 3 Tbsps.
- Vanilla – ½ tsp.
- Lemon zest – ¼ tsp.

Method

1. In a bowl, stir together sugar, mint, and strawberries. Let stand until berries are softened, about 15 minutes.

2. In a bowl, beat the remaining ingredients with a mixer for 2 minutes.
3. To assemble: scoop about 2 tbsps. ricotta mixture into each parfait glass. Top each with a large spoonful of strawberry mixture. Repeat layers.
4. Top with additional fresh mint. Serve.

Nutritional Facts Per Serving

- Calories: 159
- Fat: 6g
- Carb: 18g
- Protein: 9g

Chocolate-Date Truffles

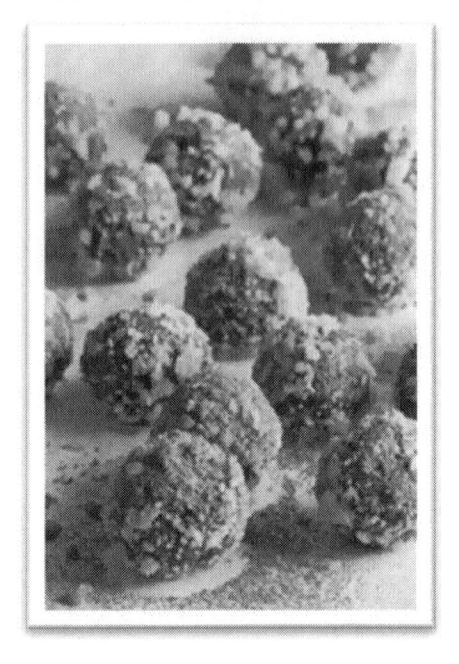

Prep time: 10 minutes	Freeze time: 1 hour	Servings: 10

Ingredients

- Coarsely chopped walnuts – ½ cup
- Salt – 1/8 tsp.
- Pitted whole Medjool dates – 1 ½ cups
- Unsweetened cocoa powder – 3 Tbsps.
- Apple juice – 1 Tbsp.
- Salt – ¼ tsp.
- Water

- Cocoa powder

Method

1. Process walnuts and 1/8 tsp. salt in a food processor until finely chopped. Transfer to a bowl.
2. Combine the next four ingredients (through ¼ tsp. salt) in the food processor. Pulse until mixture forms a thick paste. Add water if necessary.
3. For each truffle, shape 2 tsp. of the mixture into a ball. Roll balls in walnuts to coat. Chill for 15 to 20 minutes. Dust with cocoa powder.
4. Cover and chill 1 hour and serve.

Nutritional Facts Per Serving

- Calories: 105
- Fat: 4g
- Carb: 19g
- Protein: 2g

Citrus Custard

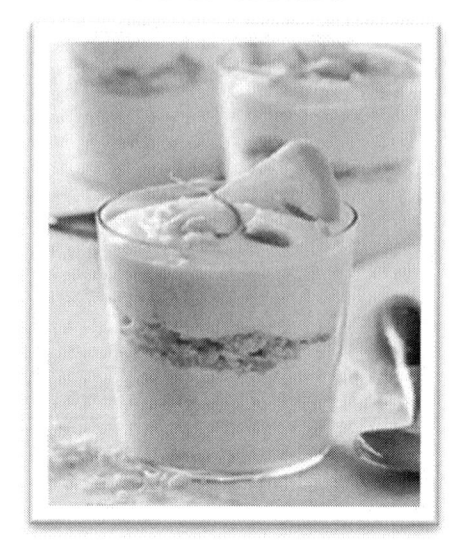

Prep time: 10 minutes	Cook time: 5 minutes	Servings: 4

Ingredients

- Sugar – ¼ cup
- Cornstarch – 2 Tbsp.
- Low fat (1%) milk – 2 ½ cups
- Egg yolks – 4, lightly beaten
- Orange zest – ½ tsp.
- Vanilla – ½ tsp.
- Coarsely crushed shortbread cookies – ¼ cup
- Orange slices

Method

1. Stir together cornstarch and sugar in a saucepan, stir in milk. Cook until thick and bubbly. Cook and stir 2 minutes more. Remove from heat.
2. Bit-by-bit, stir in about 1 cup of the hot mixture into the egg yolks. Return to saucepan. Bring just to boil and remove from heat.
3. Stir in orange zest and vanilla. Pour into a serving bowl or four dessert dishes and cover surface with plastic wrap. Cool slightly.
4. Chill at least 4 hours before serving. Do not stir.
5. Top custard with crushed cookies and orange slices.
6. Serve.

Nutritional Facts Per Serving

- Calories: 212
- Fat: 7g
- Carb: 28g
- Protein: 8g

Creamy Chocolate Pudding

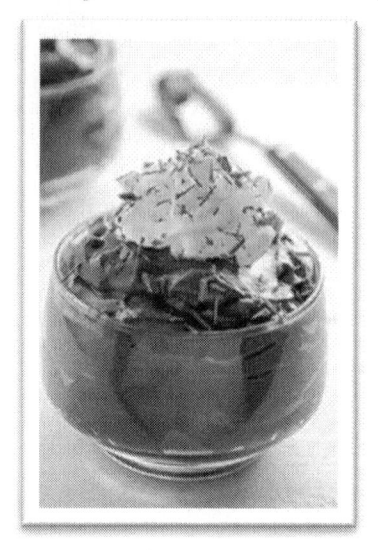

| Prep time: 5 minutes | Cook time: 0 minutes | Servings: 4 |

Ingredients

- Ripe avocado – 1, peeled and cut up
- Banana – ½, peeled and cut up
- Unsweetened cocoa powder – ½ cup
- Milk – ½ cup
- Honey – 3 to 4 Tbsps.
- Vanilla – 2 tsps.

Method

1. Combine all the ingredients in a blender. Blend until smooth. Chill and serve.

Nutritional Facts Per Serving

- Calories: 163
- Fat: 7g
- Carb: 26g
- Protein: 4g

Peanut Butter Butterscotch Bites

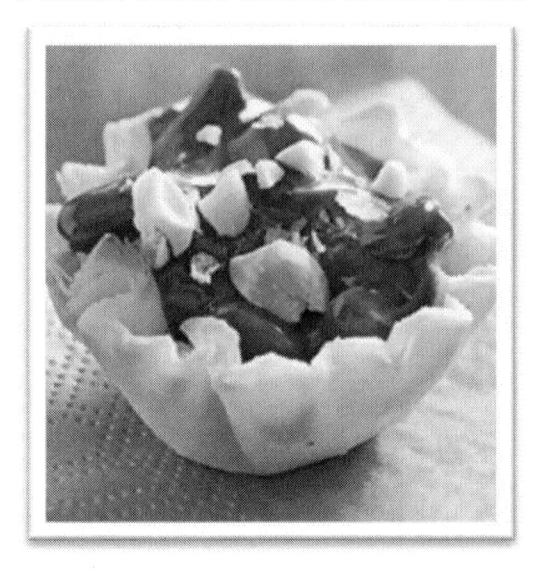

Prep time: 10 minutes	Cook time: 5 minutes	Servings: 45

Ingredients

- Semisweet chocolate pieces – 1 ¼ cups
- Butterscotch-flavor pieces – ½ cup
- Fat-free half-and-half – 1/3 cup
- Unsalted peanuts – 1 cup
- Baked miniature frozen phyllo shells -45
- Unsalted peanuts – ¼ cup, finely chopped
- Flaked sea salt

Method

1. Melt the butterscotch-flavor pieces, and chocolate pieces in a saucepan. Stirring frequently and melt until smooth. Stir in half-and-half until smooth. Stir in the 1 cup peanuts.
2. Quickly spoon peanut mixture into phyllo shells (using about 2 tsp. per shell).
3. Before mixture is set, sprinkle tops with the finely chopped peanuts and flakes sea salt.
4. Let stand at room temperature for 15 minutes and serve.

Nutritional Facts Per Serving

- Calories: 85
- Fat: 5g
- Carb: 8g
- Protein: 2g

Apricot Pocket Cookies

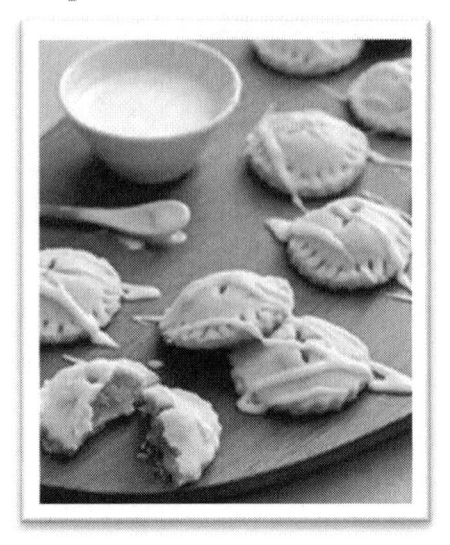

Prep time: 1 hour	Cook time: 10 minutes	Servings: 24

Ingredients

- Butter – 1/3 cup, softened
- Granulated sugar – ½ cup
- Baking powder – ¾ tsp.
- Salt – ¼ tsp.
- Light sour cream - ¼ cup
- Egg – 1
- Vanilla – 1 tsp.
- Cake four – 2 2/3 cups, sifted
- Dried apricots – ¾ cup

- Granulated sugar – 1 ½ Tbsps.
- Powdered sugar – 1 cup
- Fat-free milk – 3 to 4 tsps.
- Almond extract – 1 tsp.

Method

1. Beat butter with a mixture in a bowl for 30 seconds. Add ½ cup sugar, salt, and baking powder. Beat until combined. Add vanilla, egg, and sour cream. Beat until combined. Beat in flour. Divide dough in half. Cover and chill dough about 1 ½ hours.
2. In another bowl, combine apricots and enough boiling water to cover. Let stand for 1 hour. Drain and pat dry apricots. Finely chop. Combine apricots and 1 ½ tbsps. sugar.
3. Preheat oven to 375F.
4. Lightly flour your work surface. Roll half of the dough to 1/8 inch thick. Cut dough into rounds with a cookie cutter.
5. Arrange half the cutouts 1 inch apart on ungreased cookie sheets. Brush outer edges of cutout with water. Spoon rounded teaspoons of apricot mixture in centers of cutouts on cookie sheets. Lay remaining cutouts over filling. Lightly press edges of assembled cooking to seal.
6. Bake until firm and bottoms are lightly browned, about 8 to 9 minutes. Remove and cool on wire racks. Repeat with the remaining dough and filling.
7. For icing, in a bowl, stir together the remaining ingredients; add more milk, 1 tsp. at a time, to reach drizzling consistency.
8. Drizzle icing on cooled cookies.

Nutritional Facts Per Serving

- Calories: 132
- Fat: 3g
- Carb: 25g
- Protein: 2g

Conclusion

Diabetes can be an annoying condition with lots of limitations and risks, however, it doesn't have to be a life sentence. Awareness is the first step to making conscious change. The next step is to be determined to make a conscious change. Develop a plan and jump into action. There are several things that you can do in order to control diabetes, the most important and perhaps the most powerful one of them is modifying your dietary habits. We hope that you have found our guidance on low carb foods, foods to seek and foods to avoid helpful in your journey to combat diabetes.

Printed by Amazon Italia Logistica S.r.l.
Torrazza Piemonte (TO), Italy